To

Christopher, Alyssa, Michael

The Room
At the End of
The Universe

*True Stories
About The Struggle
Against Brain Disease*

Dr. Anthony Adamo

outskirts
press

The Room At The End Of The Universe
True Stories About The Struggle Against Brain Disease
All Rights Reserved.
Copyright © 2022 Dr. Anthony Adamo
v4.0

The opinions expressed in this manuscript are solely the opinions of the author and do not represent the opinions or thoughts of the publisher. The author has represented and warranted full ownership and/or legal right to publish all the materials in this book.

This book may not be reproduced, transmitted, or stored in whole or in part by any means, including graphic, electronic, or mechanical without the express written consent of the publisher except in the case of brief quotations embodied in critical articles and reviews.

Outskirts Press, Inc.
http://www.outskirtspress.com

ISBN: 978-1-9772-4771-1

Cover Photo © 2022 www.gettyimages.com. All rights reserved - used with permission.

Outskirts Press and the "OP" logo are trademarks belonging to Outskirts Press, Inc.

PRINTED IN THE UNITED STATES OF AMERICA

TABLE OF CONTENTS

Preface i

Cosmic Connection 1

All Cadavers Have Blue Eyes 12

Resurrecting Nina 22

The Room at the End of the Universe 31

From the Corner of My Eye 43

Conversation with A Dying Priest 50

The Girl from Babel 58

Terror Management Theory 66

The Light That Never Goes Out 75

Kaleidoscope 83

The Time Traveler 90

Reptilian Housewives 102

Cassandra's Nightmare 109

Do Helicopters Eat Their Young? 118

The Eternal Vigil 129

Anna O. Redux 135

The Premature Burial 143

The Remains	151
Man Plans…	158
Tomorrowland	166
The Palace in My Head	172
The Monster Within	178
The Banquet	188
Primun Non Nocere	194
Of Minds and Maps	200
The Carnival	206
Lost in the Fugue	210
Mrs. Goldberg's Office Visit… or	
A Fourteen-Billion-Year History of the Human Brain	216
Memories of Dreams	228
Final Greetings from Room 237	237
Afterlife	240

Acknowledgments

First and foremost, I want to thank the many patients I have diagnosed and treated especially the ones whom I have written about in these pages. To protect their confidentiality, some historical and personal details have been changed. Also, special thanks to my office manager Rose Stroehlein who provided invaluable time and patience so I could learn the intricacies of Microsoft Word. The folks at Outskirts Press, particularly Dana Nelson, helped every step of the way through the editing and publication process.

Preface

Speaking about medicine, Hippocrates once said, "The art is long, life is short." In the practice of Neurology this is even more evident. We deal with some terrible disorders and diseases afflicting the brain of which we have vast gaps in knowledge. Sometimes, in lieu of curing, all we can offer is to help the afflicted navigate a course through their adversity with simple compassion.

The patient stories compiled in this book are true. Some accounts represent compilations of more than one patient, and some details are changed to protect confidentiality. All were born out of midnight hospital consults and daytime office visits that are the staple of any medical specialty practice.

When I was a young boy, about eight years old, I would often spend time in Upstate New York's Dutchess County, where my grandparents lived. Their house sat on several acres of untouched land and, with no streetlights to be found, had a spectacularly clear view of the nighttime sky. I fancied myself a young astronomer in those days, complete with books about space, star charts, and a handy telescope. On one dark summer night, I chose to just lie down on a grassy slope near the house and stare upward. The view was majestic. I remember seeing the faint glimmer of the Milky Way arching across the sky. I could identify Mars, Jupiter, and some of the brighter stars, such as Polaris, Arcturus, and Antares (or so I proudly believed). After a while I stopped trying to play astronomer and simply gazed deeply into the vast orb of starlit darkness. In a matter of minutes, or perhaps much longer as I lost my sense of time, I felt as if I was floating and being engulfed by the infinitude of the sky above me. I lost sight of the well-lit house on my left and the tree-lined country road to my right. Frightened and awestruck, I leaped up and ran across the lawn and into the house, relieved to see my parents, grandparents, and cousins sitting in front of the TV watching an episode of *Bonanza*.

I never understood what terrified me so on that summer night so long ago. The experience of awe and wonder, sometimes referred to as numinous, is a universal human experience. It can happen when one feels something far greater than oneself like the beauty of the nighttime sky or the birth of a child. Such mysteries allow us to briefly transcend our narrow selves. Some of these feelings can occur in the cold clinical world of medicine as well. Watching fellow humans struggle with life-altering and sometimes tragic diseases with love, grace, and courage is often more than inspirational. It can be life affirming.

I believe there are lessons for all of us contained in these stories.

The journey is difficult, immense, at times impossible, yet that will not deter some of us from attempting it. We cannot know all that has happened in the past, or the reason for all these events, any more than we can with surety discern what lies ahead. We have joined the caravan, you might say; at a certain point we will travel as far as we can, but we cannot in one lifetime see all that we would like to see or learn all that we hunger to know.

Loren Eiseley, *The Immense Journey*

The world is a fine place and worth fighting for and I hate very much to leave it.

Ernest Hemingway, *For Whom the Bell Tolls*

Cosmic Connection

The universe is big, if not infinite. The observable universe is nearly 14 billion light-years in all directions. That's just about the horizon limit in which we can see the ancient light from the Big Bang. The universe is accidental. Chance and circumstance seem to govern all, even the evolution of life on earth. It's even possible, the scientists tell us, that everything began from nothing. A mere quantum fluctuation in the vacuum of space may have created the Big Bang explosion of matter and energy that gave rise to everything—galaxies, planets, people, and flowers.

The universe is temporary. The billions of stars in the billions of galaxies will eventually burn out; their nuclear furnaces will run out of energy and become black holes. Even atoms, the building blocks of everything, may become unstable and disintegrate. Everything and everyone we have ever known or will know, from my favorite pine desk where I am seated now to our loved ones, will eventually be gone without a trace.

These are the tenets of modern science. At first glance, it

seems that there is little room for joy or comfort in such harsh light. But there is some grandeur in this view of life, accurate or not. Our moments in the sun are precious and unique despite all the pain and suffering we must endure. There is tragedy and joy in all our lives, and when it all ends, who's to say what's next—an afterlife, a higher consciousness, or maybe just eternal nothingness. Kevin M., the electrical engineer who I was called to consult on during his fateful hospital admission some years back, had something to say about all of this.

The first time I met Kevin M. he was in a coma. About an hour earlier he was enjoying a backyard barbecue honoring the recent college graduation of one of his two children. In his midfifties and married for nearly thirty years, Kevin had what most of us would regard as a good life—two successful children, a stable marriage, and financial security. He was an electrical engineer who had worked for NASA and Grumman over the years. Of course, at our first encounter he could not tell me any of this. At the family picnic he suddenly broke out in a sweat and collapsed to the ground. The ER chart read "no prior medical history," and he recently had passed a complete physical by his family doctor with the exception of a mildly elevated cholesterol level and some reflux gastritis symptoms. Nonetheless, his heart suddenly went into ventricular fibrillation, a kind of rapid and erratic quivering that is usually the most lethal of all cardiac arrhythmias (and in this case was precipitated by a heart attack). He received immediate CPR by one of his houseguests, who fortuitously happened to be a trained EMS technician, and so his heart maintained a weak pulse until his arrival at the emergency room. The staff quickly intubated him to force oxygen into his lungs and placed him on a mechanical respirator while they shocked his heart back to life with a pair of charged paddles applied to his chest.

With his heart back to work and reliably pumping blood to the brain, the ER staff expected him to wake up shortly, but this was not happening and so I was called. I was half expecting this to be another dreadful case of severe irreversible coma resulting from lack of blood and oxygen to the brain—a "fried brain" as some of the medical staff jovially refer to this condition or, cloaked in more technical but less vivid parlance, hypoxic-ischemic encephalopathy.

As the days passed, Kevin appeared to struggle to regain consciousness. He became agitated, pulling at his limb restraints designed to keep him from pulling out his breathing tube. His pupils were dilated and constricted as if they were ready to erupt. He finally appeared to understand some simple verbal commands from the staff, and his eyes would tear when his wife and children visited. One evening he accomplished, on his own, what the anxious intensive care doctor was procrastinating about: he managed to contort his body in the bed just enough so his right arm could reach his face, and he pulled out the respirator tube from his throat. In a raspy voice he uttered, "Now I can go home!" and proceeded to untie his restraints. He was even well enough to undergo desperately needed heart bypass surgery a few days later with no major complications.

The fire of consciousness requires a never-ending flow of oxygen and glucose. Once interrupted, the fire quickly extinguishes. Brain death, persistent vegetative state, and permanent coma are some of the typical consequences of even just a transiently defibrillating heart or cardiac arrest. But Kevin was different. He recovered intact with no obvious behavioral or cognitive issues, so when his wife contacted me with great concern weeks after Kevin had been discharged from the hospital, I was surprised.

"He's been a little strange, different…kind of quiet which is not like him," she said.

"Well, he's been through a very traumatic experience—heart attack, coma, cardiac surgery—in the span of a few days. Has he been having any headaches, dizziness, memory issues, or any other specific complaints?" I asked.

"No, he says he feels fine. He's even back to work part-time. He spends a lot of time in his study at night. He's reading all these religious texts." Her voice quivered.

"What do you mean?" I asked.

"He was never very religious; I mean we're Catholic and we raised our kids Catholic, but we're not strict about it. We go to church on some Sundays and holidays, but we're all kind of lukewarm about religion. He's been reading all these texts—the Bible, Koran, the Torah, the Bhagavad something or other. He's positively voracious about it. I don't know what to do."

I suggested that she just keep an eye on him. He didn't sound depressed or psychotic by any means, just a little inspired or obsessed with his newfound religiosity. Sometimes we see this with catastrophic or life-threatening illness, I thought.

"It'll pass," I told his wife.

Even hardened atheists and those steeped deep in scientific materialism often find God after traumatic experiences like the loss of a loved one or a near-fatal accident or injury. Often an ordinary experience in nature can evoke mystical-type emotions. Who has not felt overwhelmed with childlike awe while gazing at a beautiful starry night sky or the vast ocean at twilight? Such experiences are universal across all cultures and creeds.

Several weeks passed before I heard from my patient's wife again. This time she was more frantic and worried.

"A couple of days ago he went into the city to catch up on some of his work. He apparently took the subway up to the Cathedral of St. John the Divine; it's on the Upper West Side and out of the way to his office. Anyway, he says he just went there and he says he got overwhelmed and got really dizzy and nearly collapsed. He ended up at St. Luke's Hospital. They checked him out and said he was fine. I picked him up and brought him home." She added that she would feel a lot better if he came in to see me.

The Cathedral of St. John the Divine was built over a century ago. It is the largest cathedral in the world with Romanesque and Gothic architectural influences. The Great Rose Window, found on the western wall, is one of the largest stained glass windows in the world. It depicts Jesus Christ surrounded by

Old and New Testament prophets. Inherent in the building's construction is a "sacred geometry" full of numerological signs and symbols specifically referring to the book of Revelation (of which St. John is considered to be the author) and its vision of the end of the world. The digits of the length (601 feet) and height (124 feet) of the cathedral add up to seven. There are seven lamps above the high altar. This is what I learned from Kevin during his office follow-up visit with me. He was very excited about the cathedral. His enthusiasm for all things religious—reading sacred texts and researching religious history—was almost infectious if it weren't so troubling. He began ignoring his family and had little interest in anything else. He thought it odd that his family and I found this all a little obsessive. In my office his wife broke down and cried. All I could do was suggest some counseling as his problem was not remotely neurological. He wasn't demented or deranged. This wasn't a psychosis or a delusion, but with his wife's insistence and my half-hearted urge to appease her, he decided to see a psychiatrist.

The psychiatrist, an older Indian gentleman who is an observant Hindu, found our patient to be charming and intellectual, if a bit curious, to his wife's chagrin. Incensed by this doctor's seemingly medical incompetence, Kevin's wife started to research the matter. Thanks to the search engines at Google, she reached a dramatic diagnosis that she was convinced I overlooked, and she was clearly exasperated over this.

"My husband has a brain tumor, and it would be located in the right temporal lobe. You obviously missed the diagnosis here, Doctor, and I only hope that it's not too late," she said casually.

She went on to inform me of some new neurologic research she had uncovered in her internet search with a supreme self-confidence in her newfound medical knowledge.

"You see, Doctor, modern neuroscientists have discovered a 'God center' in the human brain—the temporal lobes. Feelings of intense awe and religious mysticism can originate here. Joan of Arc probably had a brain tumor right there." She pointed to her right temporal area and went on to enlighten me further. "All those visions, hearing voices, mystical experiences, she was suffering from a damn tumor, and that's what my husband has…and I'd like to know what you're going to do about it, Dr. Adamo!"

The right and left temporal lobes have evolved with many crucial roles. Language, both its production and comprehension, is primarily the domain of the left temporal lobe. Memory and emotions are also the domain of the temporal lobes, including the hippocampus and amygdala Certain types of seizures (once known by the older term "temporal lobe epilepsy," where the victim will suddenly stare blankly) originate in the temporal lobes (right or left). Many patients who experience these seizures often report feelings of religious awe, mystical communion with the world as one, oceanic feelings of depersonalization, and other dramatic and ineffable sensations as an aura or prelude to the actual seizure. There had been recent speculation that perhaps the human brain has evolved as such to interpret certain experiences with the preconceived notion that God exists—an omniscient, all-powerful deity that we come in contact with as evidenced by these feelings and experiences. Perhaps then, the argument goes, the human brain is hard-wired for religion.

"Mrs. M., please listen. Your research is impressive. It is true that brain tumors often grow in the temporal lobe regions, sometimes very malignant ones which can cause seizures or strokes, but that's certainly not the case with your husband. First of all, he is not suffering from any types of seizures as far as we can tell. Also, his brain MRIs have been consistently normal with no suggestion of any tumor at all."

I almost felt bad about repudiating her theory. To her thinking, a diagnosis of a temporal lobe tumor would have been welcome. We could have the tumor cut out, and she would get her husband back intact without this religious obsession.

Kevin had a simple response to all of this: "I don't have a goddamn brain tumor. I had a heart attack and that's all!" He was not interested in fixing his problem because, as he saw it, there was no problem. He enjoyed his newfound religiosity and did not see it as alien to his character. Was this a genuine personal epiphany after suffering a life-threatening experience? Was it some kind of abnormal obsession as his wife suggested?

"Perhaps we should have psychiatry follow up with you, just for a consult. You know, after a traumatic experience like this, it is very common to suffer depression and anxiety."

He looked at me with some incredulity. "Listen, Doc, I'm

not crazy and I'm not depressed and I'm not Joan of Arc! It's just that I realize certain things now, see things a little differently now. You know what I mean?"

Several months passed. Things seemed to quiet down with Kevin. I hadn't received any frantic phone calls from his wife and no word from any local emergency rooms about my patient being admitted. Then one day he showed up during office hours for an unexpected visit. It was a slow day so my secretary put him on my schedule to be seen.

"Listen, Doc, I really don't think there's anything wrong with me. I mean, it's not like I'm some religious fanatic. It's just that things change, right? When someone goes through what I did, it changes you. How can it not?"

I could see he was tentative, kind of hesitant. He was holding back on something. "You know, your wife thinks you have a brain tumor," I said, half trying to be funny, "but I don't think that's your problem."

"I don't think I have a problem. Look, I survived for a reason, and I don't think it was just the luck of the draw. Can I tell you something? I haven't told anyone else, not even my wife."

I wasn't sure what was coming next.

"I have this memory, and I can't place exactly when or where I got it from. Maybe it was before the heart surgery or maybe after when I was still in recovery. Maybe it's from when I first collapsed and was almost dead. You know how you hear all those stories about people who almost die, and then they are revived? You know, stories about white lights and tunnels and seeing their families and dead relatives."

"Yes, I am familiar with this phenomenon; there's a fair amount of scientific literature regarding this. It could be a type of vivid dream state triggered by oxygen deprivation to the brain. They're called NDEs, near-death experiences. There are different theories about what exactly causes them." I was trying to sound comforting. I was vaguely concerned about the discussion turning mystical. Something ingrained in me and my medical training wanted to keep this all very practical, but we were both in uncharted territory here. Not your typical fifteen-minute neurology office follow-up visit. But the patient before me was not interested in scientific practicality or a tidy medical reassurance.

"I believe something real happened to me. I felt something real—a sense of peace or fulfillment. I saw my family…and the ocean, I think. But no white light, just a presence. Something… and then I remember the medics shouting over my body."

"Is this why you became so interested in religion, the cathedral, and all that?"

"I think so. I find learning about religion and God very comforting, and I'm not sure why. I know I've been worrying my wife to death."

"All right, then why don't we make a deal," I said through a smile. "I'll call your wife and explain to her that I don't believe you are suffering any kind of psychiatric disorder, and you certainly are not dying from a brain tumor, okay?"

"And what do you want me to do, Doctor?"

"Take it easy on the religion. I don't mean become a non-believer, and I'm not discrediting your experience in any way. It's a beautiful mystery, and it can be interpreted in many ways. Just ease up a little because you're driving your wife a little crazy!" We both laughed.

That was the last time I ever saw him. But I hear that every Sunday he treks into New York with his family to attend mass at St. John's.

All Cadavers Have Blue Eyes

The dissection of human cadavers for medical knowledge has a three-thousand-year history. The ancient worlds of the Greeks, Muslims, and Christians all dissected corpses, even when forbidden. Galen, Vesalius, and Da Vinci advanced our understanding of the body while fearlessly quartering and flaying the putrid and decomposing dead. Their endeavors gained much knowledge to benefit the living for all time. And, as I learned in my first year of medical school, one may learn just as much about the mind as the body from such work.

It was a world of cool stainless steel and the acrid odor of formaldehyde saturating human flesh. Most would have considered it macabre, if not repulsive, but for me it was the Promised Land, the rich reward of all my countless hours of studying and memorizing and giving up much of my college social life. This was the Gross Anatomy 101 medical school lab: day one.

A middle-aged Indian professor, a former surgeon,

admonished the class at the start: "Your cadaver was once someone's mother, brother, son, grandfather, so treat him or her as such. This collection of organs, brain, and skin, once a walking and talking person, will be dissected and mutilated by you over the next year, but never forget that it was once human like you."

Our professor, I would later learn, gave up his surgical career in his prime due to the development of an essential tremor. His once razor-steady hands started to quiver with intention. The rumor was once he nearly killed a young patient when he nicked her carotid artery during a procedure. He never operated on the living again.

At first, we were reluctant if not apprehensive to make the first incision in the freshly preserved, untouched body. Both awe and revulsion dominated our emotions. We named our cadaver, an elderly woman probably in her eighties. We were told that naming her would help humanize our situation so we would always remember exactly what we were doing: kids just out of college now playing doctor on a corpse. We argued about who would make the first cut, an abdominal incision, on the first day. The flesh was taut and boggy, and we all flinched as one of us applied the cold steel scalpel midline down the belly. Her translucent bluish eyes seemed to flinch.

The revulsion, with a vague sense that we were doing something very wrong, would soon vanish. There was a schedule to keep, anatomy lessons to be memorized, and a relentless stream of exams to pass. Soon there would not be the luxury to wonder about Lucy's former life, the name borrowed from the protagonist of the classic TV show *I Love Lucy*. We would eventually learn that unlike many of the other cadavers that were unclaimed bodies or homeless souls, institutionalized for decades and long forgotten by any kin, Lucy was donated to the medical school by her children in the name of science, to advance the education of young doctors in training like us. Were we really worthy of such nobility?

I remember after a particularly grueling dissection, my team retreated to the local diner for lunch, our appetites completely unaffected by what would have been considered a gruesome task just a few weeks before we started school. We were sitting around our table, enjoying hamburgers and fries, and talking feverishly about our work. "I took out Lucy's aorta intact; I don't think anyone else in the class managed that," one of us proudly proclaimed. "Yeah, but remember how you mangled that kidney," I retorted. We were oblivious to our surroundings until I realized that the elderly couple across the way was staring, and a mother with her two children had just changed booths to move farther away from us. Were we being callous, disrespectful? Did they think that we were a bunch of psychopaths gleefully discussing our unspeakable crimes?

Lucy would gradually lose her identity as a dead human and become a liver, an aortic artery, a tumor-filled lung. The last finding completely puzzled us. We couldn't find anything like it in our color-photograph textbook. We were appalled to discover the golf ball-size lesions in her right and left chest until our instructor reminded us, "Ladies and gentleman, your cadavers died of something; that's why they're here...so don't be surprised if you find a ruptured aorta, infarcted heart, or stroked-out brain. You're not only playing doctor; you're also playing pathologist."

At the end of the year, we would be rewarded with the brain. At this point, Lucy's body was reduced to unrecognizable debris of piecemeal organs, tissue, and skin combining into a formaldehyde-oozing translucent blob. Even her face had been dissected at this point, but not without protest. The most hardened of our young anatomists recoiled from that task. Performing splenectomies and mock cardiac surgery was one thing, but a face? That most human and unique personal aspect of our anatomy. We called over our professor, the one whose hands once failed him but seemed now uncannily steady. "I need you to remove both orbits, eyes intact, peel the facial skin over, start at the forehead." We visibly cringed.

Eventually, the hacksaw came out, complete with Black & Decker label. The skull is hard but can be cracked like an egg if you devote the time and effort. Flaps of skull were removed. The brain had to be severed from the brain stem. It felt sacrilegious at first, taking the murderous scalpel and cutting through the medulla. This would be instantly fatal if she were alive. Even now, months after the virgin incision was made, we had to remind ourselves, "She's not alive; Lucy is dead. She doesn't feel any of this."

Like the ancient art of trepanation, we would cut out the bone flaps to remove the glistening matter—gyri and sulci—folded over and over. Under the harsh fluorescent lights, the oozing brain seemed luminous. Holding a human brain in your hands, a mere three pounds, that just a few days ago was thinking and feeling, one cannot help but be astonished by the fact that a hundred billion jelly-like neurons with their hundred trillion connections somehow manage to create memory, emotion, language, a sense of personal identity, and most mysterious of all, consciousness.

We each took turns holding the greasy, neuron-packed sphere in our hands. Is this Lucy's soul or what's left of it? If not, where is her soul? Is there anything here in this lump of brain matter that could possibly be eternal and immutable?

"Her soul is eternal; the brain is merely her worldly vessel. Everything that is Lucy—her mind, personality, soul—lives on," spoke the devout believer among us, an observant Jew who ultimately became a cardiologist.

"I don't know," someone else interjected, "how can that be? All the information that made up her memories, emotions, and personality was destroyed when all these neurons died. Now her brain is just a lump of dead flesh, isn't it?" The voice of scientific skepticism spoke.

"She lives on but only in the minds of others, in the memories of others," said another, a future psychiatrist, as if to strike a humane balance between the two opposing views.

Over the next several days, we carefully deconstructed the most mysterious and complicated thing in the known universe while we ate lunch, conversed about the previous night's basketball game, and complained about all the memorization necessary for the neuroanatomy exam. But the arrogance we had developed over the past year, grown out of our familiarity with Lucy as less and less human and more a collection of anatomical parts, quickly faded. We handled her brain gingerly, cautiously, as if we could cause some damage to her if we were not careful. We avoided using the scalpel unless absolutely necessary. The brain appeared in decent condition for an eighty-year-old. There were no obvious infarctions to indicate stroke injury, but buried under the deep cortex on the right temporal lobe was a solitary, ugly black-gray mass about half a centimeter in diameter. Lucy had lung cancer, and it had obviously spread to her brain. It may have been silent in life but could have caused seizures or memory problems. Maybe none of her doctors even knew about it, but we did. We finally had an official diagnosis for our patient a month after her death: primary lung cancer with a solitary cerebral metastasis.

Several years later, as a first-year intern at a large teaching hospital, I was called to "pronounce" a patient. This strange bureaucratic-sounding nomenclature is a kind of euphemism used by hospital staff. It means that an in-patient has just died and a doctor has to officially determine this by examining the presumed deceased, speak to the family (usually on the phone and typically in the middle of the night), and filling out the all-important death certificate. (As my senior resident warned me, "There's no death without that certificate!") This honorable but dreaded chore always trickles down to the lowest man on the medical totem pole: the intern.

The patient was an eighty-four-year-old female who had advanced congestive heart failure. She had been hospitalized for several weeks and was being treated medically with diuretics, oxygen, and an array of cardiac drugs. Still, she became more and more hypoxic due to the inadequate pumping of her dying heart and, with this, more confused and lethargic until she quietly slipped into a coma and died. This patient was a DNR (do not resuscitate), so she was expected to die. No life support to be disconnected, no brain death determination, no organ donation due to her advanced age and disease. This was as natural as death can get in a large tertiary care hospital.

The protocol for a pronouncement is standard: observe for any signs of life; use your stethoscope to listen for breath and heart sounds; check pulses, pupil reactivity, and other brainstem reflexes (like gagging); also check for any voluntary or reflexive movement of limbs, and, at the time I was an intern, run a bedside EKG to make certain there is no heart rhythm. Once completed, call the next of kin and try to sound sympathetic and empathetic even though you may not be familiar with the patient and the family—not to mention that you probably resent the patient for dying in the middle of your last chance to sleep a few hours before morning rounds. Once completed, I went downstairs to an administrative office and filled out the certificate: Name: Betty Giorgano. Widowed mother of three children. First generation Italian-American. Once a seventh grade history teacher.

I did have some familiarity with this lady. Several nights prior I was called to perform a difficult phlebotomy. Elderly patients have poor veins that make it difficult for technicians to get their daily blood samples. The intern will often be called in these cases. I typically would perform a "femoral stick" in these cases: Using a large bore needle, draw blood from the femoral vein, a large hard-to-miss vein in the right and left groin, a guaranteed wellspring of blood to fill several test tubes but painful to the patient. At that time, just a few days prior to her death, she was awake enough to be somewhat talkative, though short of breath. The pain of the femoral stick must have jarred her into greater alertness.

She asked me a question. "Young man, can you answer something for me? I keep having a recurrent dream. I think it's all these damn drugs; they make you goofy."

I could see her smile, her voice just audible behind the hissing sound of the oxygen flowing through her nasal cannula. "Tell me about it," I answered.

"Well, it's summertime, or maybe early autumn. My husband, me, and my three children are all sitting in a little cabin with a fire burning in the hearth. I think we're eating dinner. It's kind of like the summer house we used to have upstate, but we sold it a few years ago when my husband died. My children, they're maybe teenagers in the dream, get up from the table and collect their things—a walking stick, a knapsack—and begin to walk outside. It's nighttime; the stars are very bright even though there is a full moon. My daughter walks across a field and travels left toward a lake. It all looks so beautiful. My youngest son heads for the woods beyond the fields, and my oldest son heads right for a path that travels up a hill. They all turn back and wave and kind of slowly vanish out of sight. I turn around and see the fire dimming; the ambers are still glowing. My husband isn't there, and I'm alone. It isn't a sad dream, but it's not a happy one either. I don't know…"

"What do you think it means?" I asked, pressing the gauze in her right groin where the needle stick was still oozing a little.

"I don't know, but I look forward to having it. It's so clear, and each night there is some little variation, but I can't always recall every detail."

I always wondered if she told anyone else about that dream, which was so vivid and realistic to her.

"Pupils fixed and dilated, no breath or heart sounds auscultated, EKG flat." I filled out the death certificate. I remember her eyes; they quickly became an opaque pale blue. I hadn't noticed if that was their natural color. Somehow, that image dredged up a long-forgotten memory. Our cadaver, Lucy, like all the cadavers in the anatomy lab, had pale blue eyes. We had speculated that with death, the cornea would become opaque and the lack of blood flow to the iris would cause depigmentation fairly rapidly, turning everyone's eye color the same hazy aquamarine, though I could never find an official pathological explanation for this. Newborn babies often have bluish eyes for a similar reason: lack of melanin pigmentation. I thought of the dimming ambers in the lucid dream of my patient. Glowing bright at first, red, then orange, and then cooling blue like the clear stars in that autumn evening sky, then dimming, gradually becoming fainter and fainter…

Resurrecting Nina

~~

The plastic crucifix above her bed told the story of a man who died at Golgotha and came back to life to save the world. The girl was young, a teenager. Her hair was matted; there was an arc of metallic sutures across the shaven right half of her head. The blinking and humming machines forced air into her lungs, fed fluid into her veins, and removed urine from her bladder all day and all night. She was restless, sometimes thrashing about, but she was alive. There was still some hope. The neurosurgeon drained the ugly clot of expanding blood that had been quickly crushing her brain. She was not brain dead; she was in a deep coma. We needed more time before we could tell how much damage there was. That's what I told her parents standing next to the machines, under the crucifix.

A few hours ago, yesterday morning, Nina was excited about the equestrian competition that was just a few days away. "Show jumping" her mother called it. It was Nina's specialty, and she was developing a pre-eminent reputation in the sport.

She had loved horses since she was a little girl. Her affluent parents were able to cultivate a childhood passion into a blossoming career. She owned a horse called Ariel, and together they had won many competitions. Now the horse was keeping a silent vigil in her barn, waiting for the girl's voice and the familiar handful of raisins she would feed her. Perhaps the horse remembered the last run across the meadow with the girl and the ugly snap of the oak tree, the red siren moving closer and closer toward the two of them.

"It was a large subdural hematoma, some epidural and subarachnoid blood too, over most of the right hemisphere. Half her cerebral cortex was crunched and the brain stem was compressed. We got her in the OR in less than half an hour after she arrived," the neurosurgeon told me.

"The craniotomy went well, no trouble with the anesthesia; now we just have to wait and see. I spoke with the parents, tried to be realistic with them—half her brain was covered in blood when she got here, so who knows what kind of recovery we'll see," he bluntly explained.

It was a beautiful morning for riding, clear and crisp. Nina and Ariel were bolting across the field and Mom was watching from the barn. They made a graceful trajectory across the grass, much like the contrail above them in the bright blue sky. Then something happened. Maybe it was the faint roar of the airplane above them, maybe a field mouse scurried across their path, but something frightened the horse. She suddenly veered left toward the outer reach of a massive oak tree. Nina saw the large, heavy branch moving closer to her. She ducked but not soon enough and not low enough. Her head snapped the branch, and she tumbled backward off the horse, falling face down. She laid silently, unable to respond to her mother's shrieking.

Her mother managed to dial 911 on her cell phone after three attempts with her trembling hand. She turned her daughter over. The contrail above her started to vaporize. The mother noticed this and will remember this odd observation. It told her that Anna had been unconscious for about a minute so far. She started CPR. She started breathing into her daughter's mouth, a mother trying to give her child a second gift of life. Nina gasped. Her mother finally knew that her daughter was still alive.

The parents stood next to the machines with the tentacles, a behemoth that kept her heart pumping and lungs filled with air as long as it held her in its clutches.

"When will she wake up?" asked the father, not realizing how optimistic the question really is.

"I don't know; the head injury was severe. Fortunately, your wife was able to revive her quickly, she was brought to the hospital in under a half an hour, and shortly afterward she had brain surgery. She is young and her brain may recover, to a degree. The brain damage in these cases can be severe and permanent. She still cannot breathe on her own without the help of the respirator," I tried to respond neutrally. I knew that every syllable, every inflection of speech, imported meaning to the parents in these kinds of situations.

The days passed on. The ICU staff—doctors, nurses, physical and respiratory therapists—each day went home to their families, but not the parents. They kept a constant vigil. They took turns sleeping overnight in the reclining hospital chair next to Nina's bed. They brought pizza and donuts for the staff. Patients would come and go in the unit; some died, and some recovered and were transferred out. The staff learned that Nina was an only child. There were fertility issues, and the parents tried for years to conceive. She was a late talker and walker but excelled in her academics. She liked Van Gogh and was a surfer.

Her friends still visited but less frequently and in smaller numbers. We best avert our eyes from too much sadness; there is misery in all lives, but some pain is incomprehensible.

Then one day, something happened. The mother noticed a motion. Her daughter reached out with her left arm, raising it toward her as if summoning the mother. This movement was different, the mother believed. It was not the usual semiconscious thrashing that is common with the delirium of the coma stricken. This seemed willed and deliberate as if Nina were calling for her mom.

"I keep having the same dream over and over, but each one is a little different; each one has its own subtle variation," the mother told the psychiatrist. Most nights she would sleep and dream fitfully on a cot next to her daughter's ICU bed. "Each night my daughter rides Ariel, but the lawn is illuminated by a full moon. In some dreams the horse suddenly veers to the right so Nina is able to duck and avoid the tree limb easily. After her ride, we go back to the house and I cook her favorite breakfast blueberry pancakes. There's a hospital respirator in the corner of the kitchen, and we laugh.

"Maybe it was the sound of the airplane engine above the field that distracted Ariel, or maybe the contrail. But what if the plane had been overhead a minute later or a minute earlier? Well, then the accident would have never happened. And what if it was just a field mouse scurrying across the horse's path that distracted her? Well, if the mouse had been moving right to left, instead of left to right, Ariel would have veered right, you know, away from the oak branch, and then Nina wouldn't have hit her head and she would be fine."

The psychiatrist was convinced that she was becoming manic in her grief, and he prescribed clonazepam to help her calm down. But Nina's mother wouldn't take the medication. She wanted the dreams to go on, each with its slight variation, some ending joyfully and some not. She looked forward to the dream world where every possible permutation of the accident, or nonaccident, could be played out. So much in life—big and small, good and bad—is born out of chance and necessity. One improbable event cascades into another, setting up the most banal or tragic consequences.

The father confided in me. He prays, but he is not a believer or at least is a doubtful one. He had fallen back on an old habit, drinking. He is independently wealthy, so at least financial concerns and hospital bills did not trouble him. He asked me if it would be better for his daughter to end quietly rather than be severely brain damaged, her personality and memories all but annihilated. I tried to reassure him; he is not a monster for wondering, and the question is a valid one. Any good parent would be prone to ask it.

One day, over two weeks after the accident, the doctors realized that Nina would sometimes takes breaths independent of the mechanical respirator to which she was still attached. They decided to extubate her—pull out the breathing tube that has been down her throat and forcing air into her lungs. When the parents visited her the next day, she was lying in her ICU bed and no longer tethered to one of the tentacles that had gripped her for weeks. She was wearing a large oxygen rebreather mask that covered most of her face. She could utter the words "Mom" and Dad" with a hoarse voice. Her eyes were brighter, and she could see.

"Do you know where you are, Nina?" I asked.

"In the hospital…there was an accident. Did someone die?"

"No, but you have been very sick, in a coma, and you had brain surgery. Do you remember what happened?" I could see that she was struggling like an explorer lost in a strange, new world, trying to reconstruct the steps that brought her here.

"Something happened; there was an accident. I don't know."

I realized that no one could have revealed the past events to her. I was the first doctor to see her after the extubation, and her parents had not yet arrived.

"Was I in a car accident?" she asked earnestly.

"No, it wasn't a car accident."

"I had brain surgery, you said." She touched the healing wound across her right scalp.

"Was it Ariel? Is she all right? I fell off of her during a ride, didn't I? I mean, I don't remember, but I think that's what happened. Right, Doctor?"

I explained to her exactly what happened. Later on I explained to the parents about traumatic brain injury. It is reassuring. I will tell them that Nina is talking and is rather coherent. Her speech is good. The left hemisphere of her brain, the language control center was spared. The injury affected the right hemisphere only. At the very least she will likely never recall the series of events leading to the accident or the accident itself and the events afterward. This retrograde and anterograde amnesia, typical after head trauma, will likely be permanent. But that is no major loss. Perhaps it is the mind's way of sparing her more turmoil.

Many weeks passed by. Her left arm and leg, weakened from the right-sided brain injury, gained strength. She learned to urinate voluntarily again. She spent two months in a physical rehabilitation hospital. The headaches and dizziness persisted, however, reminding her of the accident she will never recall, the accident that brought her here.

Six months later, one spring morning, she had an appointment to see me in my office. Her mother was with her. Her hair had grown back; the brain surgery wound was no longer visible. She was bright-eyed, cheerful, and talkative. I explained to them that this was a dramatic recovery and was not at all typical. Traumatic brain injury, often seen in young people after major car accidents, is typically devastating with permanent language, cognitive, and behavioral sequelae. But the young brain is malleable, capable of plasticity and adaptability. Her mother explained that the only difference in her daughter that she could detect was a change in personality. Nina was more extroverted now and seemed more self-confident. Nina said she was unaware of this but joked that it must be an improvement.

"Mom says I'm more social now and more talkative too. I don't know, maybe. I guess it's the new improved Nina 2.0!" She laughs.

"Do you think you'll ever ride again?" I ask her tentatively, expecting a resounding "no!" from both her and her mother.

"Oh yes! I'm hoping to have Ariel ready for the summer competitions. I couldn't imagine not riding."

I first thought that such a proclamation could only be the result of reckless youth and immaturity. How could she consider returning to this frivolous equine sport that nearly destroyed her? Didn't she realize how improbably lucky she was?

Most such accidents result in the horribly brain damaged, the permanently comatose, and the dead. Nina escaped all of this. Only someone so young could not realize the precious and tenuous grip on life we all hold on to. But without being able to express it outwardly, Nina understood just the opposite. She would climb back onto her beloved Ariel and ride across the green meadows again, passing that old oak tree and smiling at the distant horizon.

The Room at the End of the Universe

It has been said that there are no dying atheists. When confronted with adversity or impending doom, we almost instinctively fall back on the hope of an afterlife or God. The need for permanent meaning or legacy is too great. This is why our earliest Neanderthal ancestors built burial sites. The human mind cannot bear to grasp or accept nonexistence. But this basic human need may not necessarily be filled by belief in a loving God or an eternal afterlife or a ghostly soul. Sometimes the awe felt when gazing upon a child's face or the majestic nighttime sky will have to suffice. Sometimes, in the end, it's all we are granted. And maybe that should be enough.

I quickly winded through the polygon corridors of this unfamiliar hospital. The outlay kind of reminded me of *Star Trek's* Starship Enterprise—clean, white, and geometric. The nurse gestured for me to enter the next room on the right. The immediate view was disconcerting. This visit was personal, not professional, but still old habits kicked in, and I couldn't help but assess the situation as a consulting neurologist, my typical role when I find myself in a hospital. I quickly tried to size up the patient: seems alert, recognizes me with appropriate affect, smiles but looks mildly pallorous. He was sitting in one of those hospital-size recliners with IV poles flanking both sides like scepters of some weary king—nasal cannula delivering precious oxygen.

The cardiac surgeon said, "I'm glad to see you, Doctor. Let's go over a few things. The cardiac angiogram shows at least two blocked vessels, including the LAD, which seems partially blocked. The ventricular ejection fraction is kind of low. And then there's the aortic aneurysm. It's not less than 8.5 centimeters in diameter." He turned to the patient. "I'm surprised you didn't have problems much sooner."

I nodded my head in agreement although it took some effort to keep my professional stance. This was bad stuff. Most aortic aneurysms rupture before they reach that size, killing their victims in one fell swoop, usually a sudden cardiac arrest heralded by ripping chest pain. The patient he was discussing was my father, gray-haired, late eighties, but sill looking fairly robust.

Like many ominous diseases, this one announced itself with a seemingly trivial symptom: a minor occasional cough. The family doctor dutifully ordered a chest X-ray, maybe half expecting lung cancer in this former smoker of decades ago. Instead it revealed a giant bubble in the aortic arch, just at the top of the chest.

"So what does this mean?" my father asked me days later, in the first of many phone calls to me regarding the discovery. "I mean, I feel fine, but I know this thing can kill me."

"Well, Dad, you may have had this aneurysm for a long time, but it wasn't always this big. It's been growing steadily. It's life-threatening. Surgery is a good option because you're in otherwise pretty good shape for someone approaching eighty-eight." I didn't volunteer that we now knew what would eventually kill him, sooner or later. It wouldn't be cancer or a stroke; it would be his heart.

At first there was bravado. He told me he had lived a long life and was ready for whatever came next. "Next" being death or beyond, assuming there is a beyond. We'd had this discussion before. Despite our Italian Catholic heritage, we both had always been open-minded but skeptical about orthodox religions, the idea of a personal God, and the great hereafter. I clearly remember seeing the Stanley Kubrick masterpiece *2001: A Space Odyssey* with my father at the movies for the first time in the late 1960s. Just a child, but a genuine science-fiction buff, I was mesmerized.

"So, Dad, what exactly is that black slab?" I asked as we walked out of the cathedral-size movie theater.

"You mean the monolith?" he answered.

"Yeah, the monolith."

"Well, what do you think it is?"

"I think it's some kind of highly advanced alien race," I said with confidence. Really not bad for barely nine years old.

"I think you're right, son. It's some kind of big, cosmic intelligence, maybe God."

"Maybe that's what God is, Dad." That was the best I could do. I didn't have the vocabulary or intellect just yet to take the idea further, but I felt that if there was a God, then maybe it was some kind of cosmic guiding force, not a man sitting up on a throne surrounded by trumpeting angels. Many years later I would realize this was my father's view as well.

When there is a disparity between a lethal diagnosis and actual experienced symptoms, it is easy for any patient to rationalize away the bad news. My father felt fine at the time of diagnosis in mid-October. Discussions of surgery—major cardiac surgery that would involve cardiac bypass and resection of the giant aneurysm all done while on a heart-lung bypass machine—were semitheoretical at this point. "I feel fine…let's just see what happens," he'd say and then conveniently change the subject, asking me about work or the kids.

It wasn't till months later that the condition ended its silence. He experienced gradual shortness of breath, which he, and even I, mistakenly explained away as just fatigue or aggravation. "It's your mother; she gets me upset with all her worrying," he would explain. Our conversations each night on the telephone had to become briefer. His usual long-winded sentences and familiar political diatribes became shorter. Sentences became three or four words in length. Then just one or two word responses—"agreed," "yes," "sure," "maybe." Then mostly hushed, labored breathing. One afternoon he was taken to the emergency room.

The young internist was very definitive. "He may have an aortic aneurysm, but right now that's not our immediate concern. He's in congestive heart failure. Lungs are filling with fluid, and he's got pitting edema in his legs. We'll diurese him. He should improve."

My father was gasping for air at this point. He was pale and slowly asphyxiating. It was obvious and should have been obvious to me. Never trust yourself to diagnose a family member. All objectivity is lost, and any symptom can be rationalized away. Even the most honed diagnostic mind looks to avoid a bad diagnosis in a loved one. It's a basic tenet learned in med school.

While he was gasping, the medical team asked him, "You're not a DNR, are you? You want everything done, right?" It was an insensitive and inarticulately asked question but necessary at this point. He, after all, had no living will or advanced directives. Doctors don't just get sued for misdiagnosing and mistreating. Overly aggressive treatment that is deliberately forced upon a patient can win a litigation case as well. The lawyers have every bad outcome covered.

"Do everything, everything, whatever, for God's sake," he gasped.

There are no atheists in the trenches. Confronted with the prospect of oblivion, some semblance of religion is often the default position for many of us.

For many visits to the hospital afterward, I sometimes had real hesitation about seeing my father. We both knew what he was up against, and it was easier to handle over the telephone. Vulnerability and mortality are two things we often do not easily equate with our parents, even though we know them to be all too human. It was hard to imagine a world without him. No nightly conversations on the phone about the day's political events or some newsworthy science topic. I could imagine it, but was it really possible? Could events really unfold to produce that end result?

Imagining one's own death is impossible by definition. One can only imagine the process—lying in a bed, perhaps surrounded by children, spouse, and siblings if one is fortunate enough. Or lying in twisted automobile wreckage, waiting eternally for an EMS rescue crew to arrive. Envisioning the death of a loved one, a parent, spouse, or child, however unbearably painful, is certainly possible. Yet, I had some mental block with this.

The night before the heart surgery, my mother stayed in my father's room. Before they fell asleep, they watched Fox News on the TV.

I tried to turn to my objective clinician perspective in thinking about my father's medical case. As a neurologist, we deal with tragic or adverse diagnoses all the time, often in young people just starting out in life. Brain tumors, strokes, and traumatic brain injuries can strike young and old alike. An experienced physician maintains empathy and compassion but somehow must learn to curtail his sense of sadness. Without such defense mechanisms, it becomes impossible to conduct the daily business of seeing and caring for patients.

With some contrived detachment I imagined the various potential outcomes of the surgery. I came up with three primary possibilities:

1. The complex cardiac surgery is a success. He survives the operation with no major complications and eventually goes home and resumes his life.

2. The surgery is a success; however, there are neurological complications. Putting anyone, especially a man approaching ninety on a heart-lung bypass machine for several hours is fraught with danger. Stroke, coma, or other irreversible brain damage can occur. They fix his heart, but he becomes severely brain damaged. It's a fate worse than death, and my father knows it. This fear allowed him to procrastinate for months before agreeing to the surgery.

3. He doesn't survive the surgery. His last view of this world, before the general anesthesia is administered, is the harsh, bright fluorescent lights bathing him from above.

Days before the operation we talked about this. I found it too difficult to enumerate the prospects as clearly as described above, but he was aware of all of them nonetheless. He wanted to live. He was not some elderly or demented man in a state of inanition looking for death as an end to pain and suffering. Death is still the ultimate enemy. He looked at me, smiled, and paraphrased a Hemingway line, maybe that he read or heard in a movie:

"The world is a good place, even though it's in a real mess these days, and worth fighting for. I would hate to leave it, son."

It is late autumn on the Korean peninsula. The landscape is cold and barren. It is particularly rocky along the Yalu River. There is a young man who will be married and have a son in about half a decade. He is in charge of the demolition team. These soldiers are part of the Army Corp of Engineers. They roam the lonely countryside blowing up bridges and roads. The Communists from North Korea are invading, backed by the Russians. It is the Korean War. It is the Cold War. The threat of a World War III looms, as well as the fear of nuclear Armageddon. Along the countryside there are caves and crevices full of the skulls of executed Korean civilians who fell victim to the extermination campaign.

One evening the young leader is stunned by the nighttime sky. It is full of stars, thousands. The stars are brighter than any he has ever seen. He can make out the majestic arc of the Milky Way and see the myriad of star clusters that make it up. One day he will tell his young amateur astronomer son about this. It is a moment of awe and wonder.

Far behind the American GIs there is a fading campfire. Huddled around the faintly glowing embers are the frozen corpses of young children. They are the orphans who roam the countryside, searching for food. Some of the near lifeless bodies are lying face up, staring at the same starry abyss. It is their last vision.

My father told me that story years ago, maybe even before I had a family of my own. He never repeated it, and I never forgot it.

My father smiled again at me. "Tomorrow's the big day; we'll see what happens. Remember, it's always a battle, and whatever is good is always worth fighting for." I smiled back. "That's right and your life is good, definitely worth fighting for."

Being a neurologist I had a fairly vivid mental picture of what was happening two hours into this five-hour operation, but my technical understanding of the surgical process was limited. I knew he was in deep anesthesia. His chest was splayed open, and most of the blood was recirculated via the bypass device. The aorta was probably cross-clamped so the cardiac surgeon could resect the aneurysm and replace the hole with a synthetic patch, much like a hole in a piece of plumbing. The surgeon had to work efficiently and with great skill. Every minute on bypass, every minute the aorta was clamped, there was potential for brain injury. The surgeon may congratulate himself prematurely on a job well done, but sometimes the patient doesn't wake up or seizes, or a recovery room nurse notices that the patient is mute with half of his body paralyzed after he is extubated and off life support. Then panic sets in, and someone like me gets called. The neurologist is always called when something goes wrong, often terribly wrong. After all, it is the brain that is most precious and vulnerable.

In this case, the only neurologist called was me. The surgery went well, and my father did wake up. Three or four hours later, he was still lethargic but speaking coherently. I could see that he was able to move his arms and legs, his eyes moved appropriately, and he seemed to be generally aware of the situation.

"I'm still here, right?" he said earnestly or maybe with a trace of relief and sarcasm. This told me a lot about the workings of his cerebral cortex. "Seems neurologically intact, all right," I said to myself with a smile.

Over the next few days, he was able to ambulate with some assistance. A short walk down the hospital corridor was tolerated "with some fatigue and dyspnea," according to the nursing staff. He was lucid and coherent. He resumed political discussions with me around Fox News reports without missing a heartbeat, so to speak. The cardiac surgery team was optimistic. A couple of weeks of some cardiac rehab—basically gradual physical conditioning—and he'd be on his way home. Scenario number one was coming to fruition.

It was Easter Sunday, just about a week after his surgery. I drove up from Long Island and spent most of the afternoon with him in his hospital room. He was eating regularly, and the nurses were pleased with this. He had some color in his face; the gray pallor had mostly dissolved, but he still seemed weary.

"Hey, son," he said with a note of mischief, "it looks like I've been resurrected just in time for Easter!" I smiled back. We are Catholic, and despite being somewhat skeptical of all religions, we have always adhered to the basic rituals—Christmas and Easter celebrations, baptisms, communion, and confirmations.

The daylight started to fade, and my father looked tired. I had a two-hour trip back home so I prepared to leave. I drew open the window blinds to let in more of the dusky light.

"North star?" He pointed to a solitary star in the gray-blue sky that was visible through the glass.

"No, Dad," I politely corrected him, "I think that's actually the planet Mars, should be visible this time of year."

"Well, all right. But definitely can't see the Milky Way from here. Too much damn light pollution."

I kissed him on the cheek and told him I would call tomorrow.

After the long drive back home, it was a real treat to sit in my easy chair and glance at the Sunday papers though I was too tired to earnestly read them. My cell phone rang around dark. The phone identified the number as "hospital." I took in a deliberate breath. I quickly calculated the various reasons why I would be getting such a phone call at this time—a dietary concern or some minor nursing issue. Maybe they decided to send him to cardiac rehab early and he was being released in the morning. None of these made reasonable sense. There was a problem.

"Hello…Dr. Adamo?

"Yes."

The voice identified as the CCU charge nurse. "There's been a change in your father's clinical status."

I thought what an absurd statement to make. That could mean anything from…

The female voice continued, "Your father, moments ago, suddenly developed shortness of breath. He went into cardiac arrest, and he is now being coded."

I imagined the protocol. He was now surrounded by at least one physician and several nurses. Intubation with a breathing pipe was now being rammed down his throat. Chest compressions. Cracked ribs. IV epinephrine, lidocaine…until the doctor called the failed code.

Were any stars visible from his window before he coded? The question crossed my mind. I don't know why. I wanted to believe that there were and that he could see them.

The stars are brighter than any I've ever seen. You can really see the Milky Way, made up of thousands and thousands of stars across the sky.

After I hung up the phone, I finally remembered the exact Hemingway quote: "The world is a fine place and worth fighting for, and I hate very much to leave it."

From the Corner of My Eye

Photopsias and phosphenes, scintillating scotoma, and fortification spectra—the terminology is as mysterious as the conditions they describe. Most of us know these specters of the mind well enough and recognize them for what they are: some type of short circuit in the gossamer connection between eye and brain. They are the shapeless forms and cracks of light that we see in the darkness, the blobs of white light or colored zigzag lines that tell the migraine sufferer a dreaded headache is coming. Or, for the very unlucky, the sudden lightning flashes of light that forebode a retinal detachment or worse yet, a brain hemorrhage. The medical textbooks have them neatly accounted for. Terms like cortical spreading depression, neuronal synaptic hyper excitability, and visual cortex depolarization describe how the neurons of our brain sometimes miscommunicate with each other and create these apparitions. But there are those who will have none of this scientific rigmarole. For them, the experience trumps the science. For them, the real meaning lies in the vision, not the supposed rational explanations that I have often tried to offer in my white-walled office, wearing my white lab coat.

Widowed at a young fiftyish, the man's wife had succumbed to leukemia. He had never expected this. He was the one with the high cholesterol, the high-pressure executive position, and a bit of a weight issue. She was the runner and kale lover. "Go figure. Don't the statistics say I'm the one who doesn't make it?" he asked rhetorically.

"The psychiatrist recommended I see you, just to make sure, you know. He doesn't really think there's a problem, but he's not sure." He shrugged his shoulders.

"All right, then, what's been going on with you?"

"Linda, my wife, died last year. She was sick for a long time, on and off with the cancer. She made it to one of our children's college graduation, and then things went downhill from there. The bone marrow grafts didn't take…and she couldn't tolerate any more chemo either. I mean, I think I've handled it all pretty well. I've been back to work, and my daughter just started law school."

"Why have you been seeing a psychiatrist?" The question was an honest one; he didn't seem too depressed, and life seemed to be moving on for him.

"Well, it's a little difficult for me to talk about, you know. I mean, I've always been a very stable person. Shortly after Linda died, I grieved terribly, and so did the kids. But they're out of the house now and busy with school, careers…busy in their own lives. I've been alone now, except for work. Maybe that's it; I'm just not used to being alone. We were married, happily mostly, for twenty-five years."

It was clear to me that he must have been embarrassed or ashamed to talk about the reason he was referred to me. I thought I should help him along. On his insurance referral form, the reason for neurological consultation was listed as "hallucinations—r/o organic etiology." I asked him to continue.

"You know, I've never been particularly religious. I'm Jewish, and we raised our kids Jewish as well. I wouldn't call myself a devout Jew, but I pretty much follow the rules. Maybe there is an afterlife; maybe we all live on some way. Who knows, right? I mean the universe is so complex, we don't really know that much about the big questions. And I guess that's where religion comes in to play, right?" I nodded in quiet agreement.

"Well, it's like this, Doc. A couple of months after sitting Shiva, I started seeing Linda. You know, imagined I was seeing her, only in my house, never outside or in my office or anywhere else. Usually in the kitchen, or sitting on the family room sofa. Just for a second or two, you know, from the corner of…" He stopped midsentence.

"Do you recognize these as hallucinations, or do you think this is something more?"

"No, I know they're not real. I'm not even frightened or surprised by them. When it happens, it seems normal, ordinary. She's as clear as day, silent, wearing her regular clothes. As soon as I try to look directly at her, she vanishes."

"Why did you decide to see a psychiatrist?"

"I don't know. I guess I just wanted to make sure I wasn't going crazy with grief." He cracked a smile, his first since I met him.

"Well, what did the psychiatrist think? Does he think you're going nuts?" I smiled back and thought he was ready to appreciate a little levity.

"He said that sometimes a person can have a fixed delusion yet not be completely psychotic. But these aren't delusions; I mean they can't be, right? So they must be hallucinations, right? I mean, I know my wife is gone."

"Have you been having any other symptoms, such as headaches or dizziness?" I was a little bewildered here. It's not every day that a neurologist in private practice is called on to answer such metaphysical questions.

"Well, I used to suffer migraines. I would get these throbbing headaches that were nauseating, but sometimes I would first get a warning. I would see flashing lights and squiggly lines in my peripheral vision. I rarely get those headaches anymore, but sometimes I still get the flashing blobs of light, and sometimes that's when I see Linda behind the shimmering lights."

He was describing classic migraine headaches with a typical visual aura, with the exception of the otherworldly apparition. A complex visual hallucination, I thought, perhaps triggered by a misperception of the visual photopsias and scintillations he had been experiencing. A grieving mind could easily mistranslate a shimmering blob of light into the beloved image of his lost wife. I knew he really wasn't looking for medical reassurance that he was perfectly sane, nor did he want scientific rationalism to explain away his comforting visitations.

The grieving husband was seeing a ghost, a phantasm, an apparition of his beloved wife. Now we've all seen things "from the corner of the eye," the darkened periphery of our vision where shadows and shapes reside, some real and some not. The rods and cones of the retina wear thin toward the edges of sight, and the signal to noise ratio gets fuzzy. The visual cortex is left on its own to fill in the gaps with imagination. You see a familiar face that isn't there or sense a presence when there isn't one. We've all experienced this, one way or another. Years ago, when I would occasionally read in my study for a brief quiet respite from my young children, they would sometimes sneak up on me. Sometimes I would turn around and catch them even though they could be very stealthy. Other times I could swear they were hiding in the room, but I would be wrong, and disappointed. It is not only the diseased mind, damaged from a tumor or stroke or drugs, that misperceives or hallucinates. Sometimes the brain has a mind of its own. The mind constructs a map of the physical reality that it thinks is out there, but it doesn't always get it right.

Why do we see ghosts? As long as there has been civilization, humans have been haunted by the disembodied. The ancient Mesopotamians wrote about souls possessing the memories and personalities of the deceased. The Egyptian Book of the Dead is a compendium of beliefs about the afterlife. The Roman historian Plutarch wrote an account about a haunted house and the spirit of its dead owner. Christians, Jews, and Muslims have beliefs regarding the soul as a nonbiological entity, eternal and immutable, which embodies all the unique human qualities of its owner. Ultimately, belief in ghosts is a very optimistic and cherished notion—if there are ghosts, then there are souls and an afterlife as well. All is not lost in eternal oblivion. The memories, personalities, and emotions live on somehow. What could be more comforting?

My patient was indeed comforted by even the vague suggestion that perhaps his visions were not natural but rather supernatural. Maybe some figment of her remained, for real, in a darkened kitchen corner or next to the night table. Maybe. It was his psychiatrist who suggested, to the bereaved's outrage, that a temporal lobe tumor could be to blame. The fusiform gyrus, in the temporal lobe, is important for face and visual pattern recognition. Could it be that his much-anticipated spectral visitations were really the workings of devious cancer deceiving him with visions of his lost wife? I reassured him that brain tumors just don't work that way. There would be other signs and symptoms—headaches, seizures, loss of balance. I offered to send him for a brain MRI to further prove that he was not diseased, but he didn't think that was necessary. He got exactly what he came for.

Natural or supernatural, otherworldly visitor or sleight of neuron trickery, it didn't really matter to him. He was content just to experience them without explanation. In time, the visitations would become less frequent and eventually stop for good. He lamented their end but told me that maybe it was his wife's message to him that he could now carry on with his life.

Conversation with A Dying Priest

IT WAS TWO or three days before Hurricane Sandy hit Long Island. The mood was quasi-apocalyptic. Catastrophic weather doesn't normally hit these parts, so people were worried. Supermarkets were packed with frantic housewives, and canned goods were rapidly disappearing from the shelves. I had stopped at the local ShopRite to buy some jars of peanut butter—a wise choice of food stuff, I thought—for the presumptive cataclysm. I remember a lady filling her cart with no less than thirty cans of tuna. I remember thinking, "If the storm doesn't wipe her out, the mercury toxicity will." Ultimately, the weather proved to be quite destructive to many homes, especially waterfront, but few lives were lost directly from the hurricane. The vulnerability of human life becomes so evident on our delicate planet in these circumstances. A rock-solid home that stood for a century and saw three generations of families grow can literally be washed away in minutes. And such is the fragility of human life.

And so with a bag of fresh peanut butter jars in hand, I trudged on when my beeper chirped. The local hospital, situated near the bay, was getting ready to shut down in preparation for the storm and was transferring patients to other hospitals. A consult was requested on one cancer patient before he was sent via ambulance to Sloan Kettering in the city where his oncologist had been treating him. It was a fairly routine request. I needed to review his seizure medications before approving his transfer.

The patient was a seventy-two-year-old male with a diagnosis of squamous cell carcinoma of the lungs. He had been treated with a partial lung lobectomy to debulk the tumor, as well as a standard chemotherapy regimen. Despite these efforts he had already had brain metastasis with multiple lesions deep in both hemispheres. He had suffered two generalized seizures as a result of these lesions. Indeed, this is how his lung cancer was discovered. One day in the church parking lot, after a sermon, he collapsed and suffered a grand mal seizure (shaking body, incontinence, and unconsciousness for a few minutes). Four months later, he had been through an entire cancer odyssey. He had recently received cranial irradiation as well to shrink the brain tumors, and it seemed to be working, though his ultimate prognosis was not compatible with many years of life. Father McKenna would probably not survive another year.

I expected the consult to take no more than twenty minutes; after all, I was anxious to get home and prepare, or at least make believe I was preparing, for the impending hurricane. I just needed to check his seizure medications (Dilantin and Keppra) and his blood levels, maybe make a few adjustments in his dosing, and then give him my benediction that he was good to go off to Sloan Kettering.

Father McKenna was surprisingly sprightly. He looked fit and trim. No doubt some of this was the result of his cancer- and chemotherapy-related weight loss, but he looked deceptively healthy, not anorexic like so many cancer victims. His short-chopped gray hair seemed to be taking root again. His voice was strong and clear. He seemed mentally sharp, despite his multiple brain tumors, and I did not detect any of the behavioral or personality quirks that we often see in people with cerebral metastasis. There was none of the disinhibition or socially inappropriate behavior, such as rude or impertinent comments or general confusion, that is typical with the frontal lobe metastatic disease he had. He held out his hand as I introduced myself and looked me straight in the eyes.

"Hi, Doctor, I'm Father McKenna, Bill McKenna."

"Glad to meet you. The plan is to transfer you out by tomorrow for the rest of your brain radiation since it looks like the hospital will be closing for the storm."

"I know. There's a storm coming," he answered somberly.

After dispensing with the usual perfunctory neurology consult details, I reassured him that there was no reason he couldn't be transferred out. His seizures were under control, he was on low dosage steroids to reduce the swelling of his brain tumors, and he would be finishing up his treatment at a world-class cancer center.

I was ready to politely take my exit—after all this was quite routine—and I needed to get back to my peanut butter stockpile before Sandy arrived, when the priest asked me a sudden question.

"How much time do I have, Doctor Adamo?"

"Well, the transfer will take about half a day to work out, so the ambulance should bring you to Sloan by tomorrow morning," I said confidently.

"No, I wasn't asking about the transfer. I mean, how much time do *I have*?"

"Hasn't the oncologist discussed this with you? You were diagnosed months ago, right?"

"Oh yes. He was not very clear. He is trying to be optimistic, but I know survival rates are not good with brain metastasis," he said, staring at the intravenous line in his arm.

"That's right. The problem is the treatment at this point may only be palliative. Once the cancer spreads to the brain, it's likely we'll see more tumors developing. Some people can survive several years with a solitary brain met, but you have many. The chemo and radiation slow down the fire, but they can't put it out." I tried to be as clear as possible. Father McKenna was obviously a very intelligent man, and I knew I couldn't sugarcoat an answer. "You are fortunate, Father. You have your faith to draw upon. Many don't."

"Well, yes. It is comforting to a point. But looking at your own mortality has a way of provoking fear, and maybe even a little doubt with even the most rock-solid faith." He smiled at me. "Even Jesus had doubts at one point," he added as if to provide justification for expressing this sentiment to a relative stranger.

The nurse suddenly walked in and interrupted. "Doctor Adamo, Father McKenna's Dilantin level from this morning is back, 11.5. Is that all right?"

"Oh, yeah, that's perfect, no need to change the dosage," I answered, trying to get my bearings back to the medical issue at hand.

I sat down on the recliner next to the patient's bed. I sensed he had more questions. The peanut butter and the storm would have to wait.

"Father, your medication blood levels are—"

But he interrupted. "Call me Bill," he said earnestly. "Were you raised Catholic?"

"Oh yes, but I've always been a bit of a skeptic. I guess the word is 'agnostic.' Maybe there are some things humans can never know for sure."

"So what do you believe in, Doctor? I mean, other than science, of course."

"Specifically, regarding the afterlife, or human soul, or God?"

"Yes, it's all related, you know."

I was hesitant to answer. After all, I was talking to a priest, my new patient, and I didn't want to offend him with scientific skepticism and doubt. This man was dying, as we all are, but he knew his days were truly limited. Did I really want to open a Pandora's box here?

"Well, Father, to be honest, I was always skeptical of any orthodox religion. No person or organization can have a monopoly on the 'truth.'" I made air quotes above my head. "Jesus Christ, Moses, Buddha, and Socrates were all great men, but I never really believed they could be divine."

"God manifests himself throughout history *through men*," he responded.

"You believe in an afterlife, Father, the kingdom of God or heaven?"

"Yes I do," he answered quickly.

"Well, that presupposes the existence of a human soul, an eternal nonphysical entity. The brain is made up of billions of neurons, and they're definitely not eternal. The mind isn't supernatural. It's a result of the physical machinery of the brain and all its electrochemistry…billions of computations that make up memory, language, self, and consciousness."

The priest smiled. "What you just said would have been considered supernatural a thousand years ago. And a thousand years from now, it will be supplanted by knowledge that makes your current ideas seem naive and quaint at best. Science can never have all the answers, Doctor."

I answered confidently, "I think that's referred to in scientific circles as 'God of the gaps': what science can't answer we invoke God as an all-purpose explanation…but science usually fills in the gaps."

"Well, Doctor, there will always be gaps. What do you believe?" The priest smiled.

I was growing more comfortable with him, and I felt surprised that I welcomed the question. "I do believe in science. I believe that the universe evolved over billions of years and that evolution can explain the complexity of life. But our understanding of nature is just beginning to barely scratch the surface. I am a little skeptical about any ideas of a personal God, but I definitely believe there is some type of cosmic purpose or intelligence behind it all, and maybe we can never really understand it. I think one big 'purpose' of the universe is probably consciousness, self-awareness, and the development of sentient creatures like humans. Well, we might, just might, be the whole reason for everything."

"What good is a whole universe with all its wonders if there are no minds to explore it and wonder about it, right?" the priest responded.

"Exactly, though everything might just be the result of some big cosmic accident. Maybe it's all the result of chance and necessity and not the design of God, as you believe." I gently pointed my finger toward him.

He smiled. "God has a hand in all of it, and there is no room for chance. All souls will be united with him for eternity after our journey in this world ends."

I felt a twinge of envy at his confidence in this pronouncement. "You know, Father, I think everyone would take great comfort in believing that there is an afterlife. That somehow I, my personality, my memories, my experiences, and everything that makes me *me* will not be lost to eternal oblivion. Otherwise all of us, our children, our work are ultimately headed for nonexistence. That's just terrifying no matter how you cut it. Maybe the only immortality we can hope for is through our genes, our children, future generations…a little piece of me will be in them…but I hope you're right".

He smiled again, adjusted the nasal cannula that was feeding him oxygen, and took a deliberate breath. "There is always the maelstrom of doubt and darkness, but one must let faith conquer it."

I cracked a silent smile back.

When confronting possible imminent death, we all want to believe in God and afterlife. Maybe I was being too cynical. His faith was genuine and a lifetime in the making. Who am I to question it? What will I believe in when the time comes?

The nurse came in. The transfer was underway. Father McKenna would be taking an ambulance to Sloan in a couple of hours.

"Godspeed, son; I enjoyed the talk."

"It was my privilege, Father."

I started the drive back home, the plastic bag full of fresh peanut butter jars on the passenger's seat.

I need to get home. There's a storm coming.

The Girl from Babel

The Tower of Babel is a classic tale of biblical mythology. I was introduced to it long ago as a young Catholic schoolboy. In the story, humanity is living in peace and speaks a universal language that is understood by all. But one day, in an act of supreme arrogance against God, humans try to construct a tower that will reach to heaven. God foils this plan by afflicting humanity with multiple languages. With the fragmentation of speech, humans cannot understand each other and are unable to complete their epic construction project. Theologians often interpret the story as a cautionary parable against human hubris, but the story works as a metaphor on several levels. Neuroscientists can view it as a story that attempts to explain the origins of language—an original protolanguage eventually gave rise, over millennia of human culture, to the thousands of languages we have today. Sociologists may interpret it as a doomsday scenario that shows the hopelessness of the human condition. People can never really cooperate, and civilization will always falter.

Ever since I met sixteen-year-old Karen, I have developed my own personal interpretation of the tale. Without the ability to speak and understand, we become trapped in our private world of ineffable images, ideas, and emotions. Without words, we can no longer communicate and connect with our fellow humans. There can be only formless thought, unshared and forever unknown. Such was Karen's fate.

It was in her math class, eleventh grade AP Calculus, where this precociously bright teenager took to learning the symbols and equations of that wordless language. I remember thinking how painfully ironic that it was here where she lost the gift of speech. An excellent student, tall and sleek with bright blue eyes and blond hair, she was first-generation American with proud Russian parents.

Her teacher called upon her to recite an answer to a vexing problem that the class was having trouble grasping, something about a leaking tank of water and the time it would take to fill it. "Karen, how about you, any ideas?" The teacher expected a correct answer.

"Glop wat the leaked kren added yeah" was the reply from the bright, blue-eyed girl.

"Excuse me, I didn't hear that," answered the math teacher, thinking the fault was with her own hearing.

Karen starred blankly, tears pooling in her eyes.

"Finger stick-glucose 110, EKG with normal sinus rhythm, brain MRI early left MCA ischemic infarct, no hemorrhage. Urine toxicology negative…" This is what Karen heard in the hospital ER less than an hour after being asked to solve a math problem in her familiar classroom. The phrases had no meaning to her not because she was unfamiliar with medical jargon, but rather the words were mostly devoid of any import, much like a foreign language. The same demon that made gibberish of her speech also muddled her comprehension of the spoken word. She lay on the stretcher, the unforgiving fluorescent light washing over her. She was terrified.

I was summoned to see her once she was settled in the intensive care unit. The remnants of her former life—a Hello Kitty backpack, a cell phone, the clothes she wore to school that day—stuffed into a hospital hefty bag waited silently on the nightstand next to her bed. Her parents stood on the opposite side, where a second nightstand would have been placed if this were a bedroom. They were tall, thin, and stately looking. I could instantly see the family resemblance. They spoke little English. They looked vaguely European. They were Russian immigrants, and Karen was their firstborn in America.

The nurse escorted them out of the room so I could examine my new patient. She was pretty and even managed to crack a small smile. Her long, athletic body (I would later learn that she was a star soccer player) filled the length of the hospital bed. She wore a Hello Kitty wristwatch that matched her backpack.

"How are you doing, Karen?"

"Okay, I…just…can't…talk…that…well." She tried to smile again, but tears rolled down her face. "Now it…kren go next mil?"

She could understand fairly well with some limitations, that was obvious, but she could barely produce a coherent sentence with understandable syntax and meaning. And she was painfully aware of this. That sacred connection between thought and speech, first forged in the brain maybe a hundred thousand years ago, was brutally severed for Karen. The neuroanatomy of this nightmare is well known to all in my profession. In this version, a tiny sliver of blood sludge, an embolus, traveled from a small defect on one of her heart valves through the left carotid artery and lodged, with cruel indifference, deep in her left brain, destroying part of the language center. Despite her youth and vigor, she was now a victim of one of the most devastating types of stroke known, the kind that obliterated, in one way or another, the ability to break free from the confines of our private minds and explore others.

I called the parents back into the room. I explained that Karen has suffered a stroke. She was not in any immediate life-threatening danger, but damage to the brain had been done. This type of stroke produces aphasia (in her case a Broca's aphasia), or the inability to speak (and to some extent understand properly). They stared vacantly. Karen raised her arm, the left one only as the right side was weak from the stroke.

"Little English only… speak Russian mostly," the mother struggled with the words. A beautiful young stroke victim, two non-English-speaking parents, and me rambling technical jargon. All of us seemingly trapped in our own aphasic hell.

According to biblical cosmology, "in the beginning there was the word." Words are the atoms of language, and language is the raw material of thought. There were words enough in this room—gibberish words, scientific words, Russian words—and more grief than words could express.

The hospital ICU is not the typical place where young, seemingly cheerful teenagers congregate. But hordes of Karen's classmates visited daily. Even some of her teachers and a soccer coach came by. I waited a day or so for a Russian translator to finally speak to her parents in detail. A middle-aged woman from housekeeping offered help, but she only spoke Czechoslovakian, which to my inexperienced ear sounded identical to Russian, I was embarrassed to admit. The kind lady explained that Russian was an entirely different language from the Serbian languages of which Polish and Czechoslovakian were a part. One of the ICU nurses knew a little Russian, but not enough to translate a medical discussion with my patient's parents. Even Karen knew Russian, but English was her primary language, having been born and raised in suburban New York. The aphasia from her left hemispheric stroke damaged her Russian language capacity just as much as, if not more than, her English capacity.

Over the next few days, Karen became increasingly somber and tearful. On my brief visits with her, she would force a smile and appear stoic, but the nurses would often find her sobbing into her pillow. I was finally able to meet with a family relative who was able to provide some Russian-English translation. I sat down with the parents in the ICU conference room, a clean and brightly lit room usually reserved for condolences.

"The stroke affected her left brain, the speech center. Hopefully, this will never happen again. She will take a blood thinner medication from now on to prevent future strokes."

Just as I finished, the translator began in their native tongue. The parents looked puzzled. "Yes, but what will happen to Karen? Will she recover; will she be normal again?" they hesitated to ask.

"She is young, and young brains can recover better than yours or mine. She will need lots of speech therapy, and time. No one can say for sure." Remember, I thought, emphasize optimism. Tell them she survived a stroke; tell them it could have been much worse. Tell them to be grateful.

Each day she struggled. She agonized over each word. The speech therapist told me she had never seen such perseverance. Once home, she worked with several tutors. She was not yet ready to return to school, but her math and science studies excelled with home tutoring. She glided through physics and calculus just as before. Equations and numbers posed no challenge, but words were slower to capture. Two months after the stroke, she returned to my office with her parents.

"Things are better. I'm back at school. My reading is slower, but I aced my math and physics midterms," she beamed. "My right-hand strength is almost normal too. After all this I'm convinced of one thing for sure."

"What's that, Karen?"

She answered slowly but clearly and with purpose. "I'm definitely going to become…either…a… computer scientist or a…math professor. I was…always more…comfortable with numbers and…equations than with words, especially now." She smiled again.

I smiled back. "Well, you know what Galileo said: math is the language of nature, the secret code of the universe. And that's always been your favorite language anyway."

Human language—the adjective is unnecessary, for no other species on the planet can make claim to this unique talent—allows for the written and spoken communication of an infinite number of ideas using streams of sounds and symbols. It is incredibly complex. The most powerful computers in the world cannot generate the language that an ordinary three-year-old makes with carefree effort. How can this be? Honeybees have a tail-wagging dance that conveys the location of a food source. Vervet monkeys have different alarm calls to warn their colleagues about incoming predators. Birds and whales have lyrical songs to attract mates and find food. But all of this pales before the symbol spinner who gazes at the stars and writes of love and loss.

Slowly, over eons of time, language must have evolved by slow, stepwise gradations. Humans and chimpanzees evolved from a common ancestor around six million years ago. We,

Homo sapiens, have been on earth for about two hundred thousand years now. In that immense journey, hominid shrieks, like the coarse sounds made by the earliest ape millions of years ago, have evolved into the words of Homer and Shakespeare.

Packing a hundred billion neurons into a small spherical skull results in several wondrous human abilities like consciousness, memory, imagination, and, of course, language. It is the firing patterns of millions of neurons, each with its own faint voice, that together conjure up the spoken words that cross the lonely gulf from one mind to another.

Terror Management Theory

~~~

It has been said that the idea of death haunts us like no other animal. After all, it may be humans alone—on the evolutionary tree of life—that possess self-awareness, deep-rooted emotions, and the desire to achieve more than just daily survival. All of civilization's greatest achievements, from the pyramids of ancient Egypt to the spacecrafts that we hurl into the interstellar night, can be viewed as epic attempts to overcome or deny the inevitability of our demise. So it is with the great societies throughout the ages, and so it is with ordinary men.

He spoke about the glaciers of Norway, having just returned with his wife, Cindy, from a hastily scheduled ocean cruise. The vacation in him was still fresh, and he spoke feverishly about it.

"I've never seen anything so white. The glaciers up there are blindingly white. So pure, like giant crystals." He showed me some photos on his iPhone.

"Yeah, they really are white, not like New York City snow that turns to toxic sludge in a day," I joked.

"It has to do with the geological process or something; the old snow constantly gets replaced with fresh new white snow. That's how the glaciers can last thousands of years. They can go on forever, barring global warming or a nuclear war!"

This was Gary's third or fourth visit to my office. In his midforties, he was a successful financial advisor who enjoyed life. With three children away at college, this vacation cruise was a sort of gift to his wife, acknowledging these landmarks in their life together. He was thinking of buying a convertible too—something sporty but affordable, maybe a Mazda Miata. "It's fast and agile, just like me," he'd say and laugh with that thunderous roar that was his hallmark among friends and family. The irony being that he was neither fast nor agile though he used to be. In his college days, he played lacrosse and was good at it. His athletic skills got him nearly a full ride at a state school, and he was proud of that, even decades later. His son played in high school and recently had joined a lacrosse club in college, but he wasn't interested in varsity. Still, Gary was grateful. Tall but no longer athletic, he took solace in the fact that at least his flesh and blood carried on some sports tradition.

He usually told a joke or two before the end of his office visit, typically something racy but not vulgar. He limped away on his crutches, having sprained his ankle recently from a slip and fall negotiating his stairwell at home.

Several days later he gave me a call. He said he was thinking of retiring. He explained that from a financial point of view, it was definitely feasible. He could sell his financial consulting business and have complete security. All three of the kids were in college, and there were more than adequate funds for them. I remember explaining to him that he needed to be fairly certain that he could find something meaningful to fill the enormous gap in time and activity that retirement would leave him with. He didn't think that would be a problem.

He had been golfing with a friend the previous autumn. Gary noticed a momentary stiffness of the right hand that would occur periodically during and after a swing. "A momentary loss of muscular coordination," he would say with a smile—apparently, I thought, mimicking a famous line uttered by Jack Nicholson in the classic horror film *The Shining*. But the real problem, the one that finally compelled him to see me, was his stiff left leg. "I feel like I'm dragging it. It's stiff and heavy." He had been recently diagnosed with a lower-back herniated disc by his family doctor and assumed this was the problem, but he knew better. Something was not right, and he was worried.

"When did this first start?" I asked nonchalantly.

"About a year ago but I ignored it. I got some physical therapy, massage therapy too, and it seemed to help for a little while. My family doc got an MRI that showed a small herniated disc. He said that was the problem, but it isn't going away."

I asked him about other symptoms—incontinence, muscle twitching, numbness, and a litany of other neurological symptoms. None were relevant to him.

He underwent the standard evaluation for such a presentation. I referred him for spine and brain MRI studies, all of which were normal, as well as some routine blood tests, also all normal. Nonetheless, his leg was stiff with abnormally brisk reflexes. He was worried because he could see that I was.

I scheduled him for an EMG study (a neurological test, this is a specialized office procedure that involves placing a small needle electrode into various arm and leg muscles to evaluate any abnormal electrical activity indicating neuromuscular disease). He said he would make an appointment but was busy now between his business and trying to get in as much golf as possible.

Months went by and I hadn't heard from my patient. I called him, wondering if perhaps he got a second opinion or transferred his care to another neurologist. I spoke with his wife.

"He's away golfing, North Carolina, and when he returns, we probably will be taking another ocean cruise—this time the Caribbean," she said blithely.

"All right, but could you have him give me a call in between vacations?" I forced a chuckle, although the whole situation seemed a little frantic to me. No official diagnosis had been made, yet he seemed completely disinterested. We talked about the likely diagnosis of ALS (also know as motor neuron disease), a progressive neurodegenerative disease usually fatal three or four years after the onset of symptoms. I did think it odd, however, that in the midst of a possible ominous diagnosis he decided to go on a vacationing and golf spree.

It was about a week later that I got a phone call from the wife telling me that the Caribbean cruise was on hold. Gary returned from his golf tournament and had suffered a fall on the course, resulting in a fractured ankle, and had undergone orthopedic surgery to fix it. He was waddling around now with a cane, and she said he was miserable.

A month later he was already scheduling his next excursion: big game fishing in Florida on his buddy's Huckins yacht.

"Gary, you know you should make arrangements, as we all should, now while you're in decent shape. A living will or advanced directives if you become incapacitated. This is the time," I explained gently. End-stage ALS results in complete debilitation of the body, usually near paralysis, but the mind is typically completely intact. A person may be completely bed stricken but intellectually sharp as ever. Think of the great astrophysicist Stephen Hawkins. He used a flicker of his thumb or eye movements to communicate his lectures and equations to graduate students, who would painstakingly decipher every word. He was too weak toward the end to even speak. And he was quite lucky, beating the odds and living for decades with this diagnosis.

"Cindy has got that all planned. Don't keep me alive if I'm a vegetable. But then again, don't kill me off too soon to collect the life insurance money." His intention was to be humorous, but his eyes glistened.

He did indeed rush off to Florida, and he returned with some spectacular "fish stories." Despite waddling around with his fractured ankle, he caught striped bass and a hefty mahi-mahi.

A few weeks went by and things were quiet. I assumed he was taking it easy, perhaps tying up loose ends of the sale of his financial business. His wife called me one afternoon. She was anxious, holding back from sobbing.

"He's been having nightmares. He wakes up in a cold sweat, says he doesn't know why. He says he can't breathe, but he doesn't seem short of breath. One night, at three in the morning, he ran to his laptop." She started sobbing. "He's planned this ten-country trip; he calls it 'ten countries in twenty days,' and he's already booking hotel rooms all over goddamn Europe!" She was hysterical. "What is he trying to prove?"

I didn't have an answer for her.

We humans have a Cassandra-like gift that is both a blessing and a burden. We are not only self-aware sentient beings, but we also carry with us the acute understanding of our own mortality. We know we are going to die, as inconceivable as that idea is. One day we will be no longer—nonexistence, oblivion—notwithstanding the comforting notions of an eternal soul and afterlife. Some of us may be blessed with faith (or delusional optimism, a cynic would argue) in these beliefs, but others are skeptical and have trouble convincing themselves of their validity under the gaze of scientific scrutiny. The sun will rise and set, our descendants will walk the earth, science will advance, wars may be fought, and humans will continue to do wonderful and terrible things, but at some point—relatively soon—you and I will no longer be part of the story. It can be quite discouraging if not downright terrifying. My father died a year before he could see my children enter college and vote for the next president, all things he was eager to experience but never will. What else will he miss out on during the next ten, fifty, hundred, thousand, million years?

Religion offers solace. That is where its power lies. Those with faith can rest easy knowing that death is the great leveler and that eternal oblivion does not await them.

Some of us turn to science for hope. Perhaps that is where any hope for eternal life resides. One day we may cure mortality like a disease. The idea of uploading our minds—personality, memories, and consciousness—onto a permanent body (e.g., a cyborg) has gained popularity with the advent of artificial intelligence (AI). Maybe someday these will be genuine prospects for humanity. But there are many of us who would claim that such faith, whether it is placed in science or religion, is a delusion with no realistic basis—a mere superstition or fairy tale that we must adopt to cope with the psychological turmoil that tries to reconcile our desire to live with the realization that death is inevitable.

Terror management theory (TMT) is the pedantic name that academic psychologists have given to this dilemma. We must reconcile our basic desire to live with the full awareness that our death is, heaven and AI notwithstanding, inevitable. This inherent conflict, present in all humans, is the wellspring of all cultural/religious beliefs, national identity, posterity, and the pursuit of science and technology—all of which are designed to deny or somehow overcome the finality of death as our inevitable destiny. We are all trying to "manage terror" in our own ways. Accordingly, then, we procreate, raise children, take vacations, find inspiration in sports and art, and work to achieve financial success to compensate for the inevitable oblivion that awaits us. As a society, we build pyramids and skyscrapers, create nations and governments, and advance technology and scientific discovery to create some permanence in a world of evanescence. We build libraries, once papyrus and cuneiform, then paper, and now digital to store the knowledge of our accomplishments. We hope this will create a legacy—if not for individuals, then as a society and as a species. But nothing is immutable or eternal, and even the universe may one day end. On that last day in an unimaginably remote future, will everything be obliterated in one giant black hole? Will the story somehow continue?

Seems like there's plenty of terror to go around for all of us.

My patient recently called me. He took my suggestion and followed up with a leading neurologist at a prestigious university medical center in Manhattan. The visit did not go well.

"He told me what I kind of already know." Gary forced a laugh on the telephone. "Things got a little worse over the past few months, more stiffness and lots of twitching in the arms now. Look, what am I gonna do?" he added rhetorically, his voice cracking.

"Plan for the worst and hope for the best" was my default statement in situations like this. I wish I could have come up with something more enlightening, and this disappointed me.

And then, his voice lifted again and seemed lighter. "I already booked my European tour," he chuckled. "I'm taking Cindy on a big trip—Italy, Spain, France. I think I should do it while I still have the stamina. Cindy was reluctant, but she's ready now. I'll send you some postcards!"

"Sounds great, just don't overdo it. Avoid the heat, and make sure you get enough rest each day and…" I replied but finally stopped. I didn't want to sound like an overbearing doctor.

Terror management theory—is that what this really is all about? I thought. Let him have his day in the sun; it's the best any of us can ever hope for.

The Light That Never Goes Out

Much has been said about the last words of the dying. From the "Rosebud" of *Citizen Kane* fame to Steven Job's reported last utterance of "Oh, wow, wow…"

The living often ascribe a vast array of meanings to these enigmatic phrases, some religious, some more banal, but always fraught with largely unknowable intent.

We rarely give similar attention to the last visions of the dying. This, in part, is the result of logistical technicalities. Dying people are often in no state to communicate coherently what they are experiencing, and they typically are in no state to discuss their experience once it is complete. Occasionally, however, people report penultimate dreams or visions to doctors or nurses. Such last dreams often embody one of several themes—reuniting with a loved one or repairing a broken relationship. It's as if the mind wants to rewrite the narrative of its owner but this time getting the plot right, the way things should have turned out and not the way they did turn out. Or maybe the mind is telling us just how things may eventually turn out.

Kevor was close to sixty years old. The hospital admitting sheet, which typically contains standard demographic and personal information like next of kin, marital status, and insurance coverage, was mostly blank. A neighbor had apparently called 911 when they noticed some odd behavior: he was attempting to mow his lawn on this cold day in January where at least four inches of newly fallen snow covered most home properties in the area. Originally he was brought in to the ER as a possible psychiatric admission. But after interviewing him, the medical staff considered him reasonable enough to warrant a neurology consult. "He just seems a little slow, a little off, but he's not delusional or psychotic by any measure," explained the medical resident to me. "His brain CT looks okay, but something's going on with him," he continued. "Come in and take a look at him when you have a chance." I remember wondering if there could be some ingenious strategy the man had in mind with his lawnmower, perhaps to grind up the snow to make it easier to shovel. Why did they drag this poor man into the hospital?

Jamaican by birth, lean and slight in figure but tall, he spoke perfect English, but his accent was unmistakable. He lived alone and owned two successful convenience stores. His parents died when he was a younger man, his mother from breast cancer and his father in a boating accident. He had one sister who still lived in Jamaica with her family. He had two children, one in graduate school and one married and working, both in their midtwenties. Though not formally divorced, he had been separated from his wife for many years. She and the children moved out and into her parents' house when the kids were just entering their teens. He spoke proudly about his children but was pensive about his life in general.

"I've been on my own. Never thought to remarry because I have a wife. Just been apart for nearly two decades. I work fourteen, eighteen hour days with the two 7-Eleven's, so the time flies by."

I looked down at the chart as I listened: brain CT normal, glucose and electrolytes normal, but his liver function tests were mildly elevated.

"Are you a drinking man?" I asked. Elevated liver enzymes often mean alcohol-related liver disease.

"No, not any more. I drank pretty regularly years ago. Ginger beer, rum. I could finish off a six-pack or two pretty readily after the kids went to bed. Wife never liked that. She took the kids, ran to her mom and dad's."

"Have you been drinking at all lately?" I asked quizzically, even though his urine drug screen and serum alcohol level were all negative.

"No, not at all. The ginger beer I drink these days is the soda pop kind."

"I ask, Kevor, because apparently you've been exhibiting

some odd behavior. You seem perfectly reasonable now, but you scared your neighbors today by trying to mow your lawn in nearly half a foot of snow. When EMS arrived, you appeared confused and disoriented. What do you have to say about that?"

"I don't know. I woke up and just thought that I hadn't taken care of the lawn in a while. I started to realize it didn't make sense, mowing the lawn in the dead of winter, after I was outside for a while. But I figured I'd get the job done anyway once I cranked up the mower. I know it doesn't make sense."

His face grew thin and his dark skin seemed to turn ashen. He stared straight through me. I thought he might be about to have a seizure, but he broke the spell and spoke again.

"I've suffered with some sadness over the years. I'm a God-fearing man, and having my family break apart was always tough. I worked hard to keep my business going, and that's what kept *me* going." The color seemed to come back into his face.

"I've been getting a lot of headaches; I wake up with them," he continued, talking more rapidly, "and I wake up a lot with them with bright light shining in my eyes."

Maybe classic migraine, I thought, with the visual photopsias and scotomas that can occur as a prelude to the headache. No, that diagnosis didn't fit. Too old, migraine is a malady of the young. Maybe he was having seizures, so-called complex partial seizures, where a person can stare blankly but still give the illusion of awareness. I decided to schedule him for a brain MRI that would provide more detail than the CT. I didn't expect to find anything dramatic.

"You should take a look at this; it's very impressive," the radiologist gleefully told me over the phone. Doctors often may have an emotional disconnect that enables them to appreciate fascinating pathology without, at least temporarily, recognizing the human tragedy that will follow as a result of such disease. Kevor's brain lit up on the MRI images once the gadolinium dye was given. Tumor was everywhere, and it was virtually hidden on the cruder CT. Both cerebral hemispheres showed infiltration of some kind of tumor. My mind started to race. He would need a brain biopsy. Was it cerebral lymphoma? Perhaps the dreaded glioblastoma multiforme- that most malignant of all brain tumors? Metastasis from a liver or lung cancer? Or maybe some weird infection? Cryptococcus? Histoplasmosis? Maybe there would be hope for him if this was some treatable bacterial disease. A brain full of cancer, though, spelled certain doom.

"Neurosurgery tells me the brain biopsy will be done next week," I explained. I tried to be as optimistic as possible. I lectured on about tumor resection, radiation, chemotherapy, and maybe just antibiotics if this was some kind of infection. But he realized the truth. Whatever this was, it would result, sooner or later, in his death.

The night before the brain biopsy I got a call from one of the floor nurses. Kevor was having trouble sleeping and asked if it would be safe to prescribe him a mild sedative. There was nothing surprising about this. A little insomnia is certainly expected hours before you're about to have your skull cracked open so a brain surgeon can scoop out tumor from your head while taking away memories and knowledge along with the disease. I called in a dose of zolpidem, a standard sedative-hypnotic, and he slept most of the night.

By the second day post-op, Kevor was sitting up and eating. There were no obvious changes in his behavior, memory, or language ability despite the fact that the neurosurgeon debulked about half a pound of tumor from his brain. He said he felt better, too. "My vision seems clearer now," he proclaimed, "and I think the headaches have stopped." I thought skeptically that his subjective improvement was probably from the steroids he was on to reduce brain swelling. Steroids like prednisone can often work as mood elevators, sometimes even making people manic with energy. I hated to break his mood of optimism, but I needed to tell him the facts, especially with his two children sitting bedside. They were well-dressed, tall, and somber. They were showing their dad some photos on their cell phones when I interrupted the visit.

"The surgeon could only remove part of the tumor, and the pathologist was very clear on the diagnosis. Remember, we talked about this. GBM (glioblastoma multiforme) is highly malignant. It infiltrates the brain with multiple extensions. He can only remove so much brain tissue without causing major damage. Next, we will have the neuro-oncologist talk to you about a chemotherapy and radiation program. That's the next step."

The survival rate for a large majority of people with this tumor is about a year. Current chemo and radiation regimens barely extend that time. The prognosis for glioblastoma is, as we often say, dismal. With rare exceptions, if any, it's a death sentence.

"We talked about this, Kevor. We know what we're up against."

His daughter reached for his hand. He smiled.

The original plan was to discharge him and have him start outpatient treatment, but he started having seizures shortly after the surgery. A visiting friend was the first to notice that Kevor was staring blankly, with eye fluttering and stuttering, and he alerted the staff. Kevor was placed on seizure medicine. The spells stopped. His face became bloated from the steroids. He wasn't going home.

One late evening, while I hurriedly checked in on him as I rushed through rounds, he looked particularly troubled and asked if he could tell me something.

"Sure, Kevor." I sat down in one of the hospital chairs next to his bed. He could tell that I was in a hurry. "It's all right, Kevor. Take your time." Despite the steroids and seizure medicine he remained quick-witted but had slowed down a bit.

"I've been seeing things, you know, visions. Colored stars, white stars—they flash and move, especially at night. I think they're the lost souls of my ancestors. Parents, grandparents, waiting for me. They know I'll be ready for them soon."

"You mean waiting for you in heaven?" I asked quietly.

"Yeah, in the next world…"

Photopsias, scotomas, visual auras—I knew these were all neuro-opthamologic phenomena, flashing blobs of light or shimmering spectra. Certainly this could be the result of the glioma affecting parts of his visual cortex, causing random synaptic firing that resulted in these unformed hallucinations. Kevor would hear none of this. He *knew* what this was. It was a cosmic event, not some electrochemical mishap.

After a week of cranial radiation therapy and steroids, he weakened. He was transferred to the ICU in anticipation of further decline—seizures, stroke, coma. Each night he said the lights got brighter, less fleeting. He said he welcomed them and anticipated their arrival regularly. He called them "heaven's fireworks."

The next morning on my rounds, his room was empty. He had gone into brief cardiac arrest, seized, and died the previous night. A couple of hours before that, he had asked the nurse to turn down the harsh fluorescent lights glaring in his room so he could see his fireworks more clearly.

Kaleidoscope

___

She was a little girl, eight or nine. I was assigned to her during my pediatric neurology rotation in residency. She had dark-brown hair and eyes, and was small for her age. Her name was Sarah. I read her index card—this was long before electronic medical records became standard at hospitals—that a medical student who was part of our ward team provided me:

> Nine-year-old female. S/P craniotomy and resection of medulloblastoma nine months ago with cranial RT and Vincristine six months ago. Admitted with headache, brain CT with some hydrocephalus. NS and oncology on case. Decadron, day two.

"Hi, I'm Dr. Adamo, one of the neurology residents assigned to you. I'll be making rounds with the neurology and neurosurgery team every day. Just wanted to stop in and say hello. How are you feeling?" I wondered if I was sounding too adult for a nine-year-old. At this point in my life, I had neither a wife nor children, so I wasn't accustomed to talking to children, sick or otherwise.

She smiled, her face somewhat swollen from the steroids she was taking to help shrink the dangerous brain swelling caused by the tumor. "Nice to meet you, Dr. Adamooo!" Her mood seemed somewhat elated for a girl struggling with a malignant brain tumor, missing school, and now with a major setback. I wondered if this could be the effect of the steroids, which can play havoc with emotions and mood, causing ups and downs, elation, and depression. Or perhaps it was just the natural exuberance of a child.

"I know what's going on, and I know it's bad. My parents make believe that I don't know, but I do," she responded, this time convincing me this was really her and not a drug effect.

As I talked to her, I glanced at the index card. Sarah had undergone brain surgery to remove the medulloblastoma after she presented with headaches and ataxia (unsteadiness in her gait) for several weeks. She had already received chemotherapy, and now radiation therapy was being considered as well. In less than a year the tumor was growing back, and she was symptomatic, prompting the readmission to the neurology ward. This medulloblastoma was particularly aggressive. In general, these tumors are bad. They grow near the brain stem and can compromise vital functions such as the regulation of breathing and heart rate. They can be surgically removed but often regrow and infiltrate the brain. Long-term survival rates are not good, even with toxic radiation and chemotherapy.

"The steroids made my headache go away," she told me as if anticipating my next question.

"That's good. Do you miss school? You might be here for a few days more, you know."

"I know, my parents might get me a tutor so I can keep up." She reached over and pulled open the night table drawer. She took out a cylinder, about a foot long, painted gold. It looked like a child's telescope. "Wanna take a look at my kaleidoscope? It's very old; it was my grandmother's. I always take it with me to the hospital."

"Thanks." I smiled and took it gingerly in my hands.

"Point it up to the light toward the window and turn," she instructed me. "It's beautiful; I can look at it for hours!"

I followed her instructions. The last time I had viewed a kaleidoscope I probably had been about Sarah's age. I turned the weighty cylinder and watched the geometric patterns unfold. It was as hypnotic as I remembered it being in childhood. Unfolding symmetrical shapes constantly appear and then transform with vivid colors of blue, green, red, and yellow, ever shifting, appearing and dissolving, exploding and collapsing.

The neurology attending spoke bluntly as he peered into Sarah's eyes with his opthalmoscope. "Blurred disk margins, swollen cups, no venous pulsation, maybe even some petechial hemorrhages, looks angry. Perfect example of textbook papilledema. You should each take a look; it doesn't get any more classic than this."

He was referring to the swelling of Sarah's optic nerves, something we could observe bedside with a basic ophthalmoscope. Her brain was swelling like an overinflated balloon because the brain tumor was taking up room in her skull, and there is little room to spare in a human head. That increase in pressure was causing the optic nerves to swell up.

"How's your vision, Sarah?" the attending asked sternly.

"I think it's okay. Sometimes it gets a little hazy, just for a second or two."

The attending was impressed that her symptoms were not more dramatic. It's amazing how resilient a young brain and body can be, up to a point.

In the days that followed, Sarah's vision did deteriorate and the headaches came back with a vengeance. The steroids could help to an extent, but without them she probably would have been worse.

A week or two went by. Patients on the neurology ward came and went, but she remained. Mom was always bedside, a couple of school friends would occasionally stop by, and a school tutor came in twice a week.

One day I made an unplanned visit to Sarah late in the afternoon. The phlebotomist had difficulty obtaining a blood sample, so I was asked to try. Her grandmother was sitting next to her. She was peering through the kaleidoscope.

"Sarah cherishes that antique; she even let me look through

it a few times," I said, looking at both of them and noticing the family resemblance.

"It's very old like me, but unlike me it still works perfectly and beautifully." She smiled and continued, "I used to listen to music, the opera especially, all the time, but with my bad hearing it's hard these days so I look forward to using Sarah's kaleidoscope. My eyes are better than my hearing so I can still enjoy it."

"Besides, Grandma-ma," Sarah interrupted, "you always say that the kaleidoscope is more beautiful than all the songs in the world, right?"

"*You're* more beautiful than all the songs in the world, my dear," Grandma-ma uttered as she looked through the scope and pointed it toward her granddaughter.

I tied the tourniquet to Sarah's arm and began searching for a good vein.

Over the next few days I learned that Sarah had an older brother just starting high school. Despite the age difference, they were close. Mom was a stay-at-home housewife, and Dad was an accountant. Grandma-ma's husband had died in a Nazi concentration camp. Sarah liked Milky Way bars, and her parents would sometimes bring her the giant-sized ones. She was an "A" student. Her first symptom of the brain tumor was heralded at school when she had a dizzy spell in gym. She kept toppling over as she was trying to tie her sneaker shoelace.

One day the neurosurgeon put up her most recent MRIs on the big screen at grand rounds. The tumor looked monstrous, bigger than Sarah on the projection. He spoke definitively: "The edema is getting worse despite the steroids, and the mass has grown about two centimeters since the first craniotomy. We're going to have to debulk it. It's one of the most aggressive pediatric tumors I've encountered, so there is significant morbidity/mortality here. I put her on the OR schedule for tomorrow morning."

That night I was on call. I had to draw some follow-up labs for Sarah, so I paid her a visit.

She was a little drowsy, probably from both the medications and the effects of the expanding brain tumor. She didn't at all seem anxious about the impending surgery. Her mom was sitting on a cot; Dad was home with her brother.

"Wanna take another look at the scope?" She smiled.

I sat on the foot of the bed and turned toward the bedside lamp. With one eye I could see Sarah's cherubic, swollen face; the other eye focused through the kaleidoscope. Once again, the beautiful geometric patterns unfolded, made up of triangles and polygons. There are an infinite number of variations and shapes that can be generated by this simple optical device. Little mirrors reflecting upon mirrors inside the scope generate fractal-like patterns that may never again be replicated with each turn of the cylinder. So, in a way, you're glimpsing the infinite and eternal. The generation of the patterns is governed by the same mathematical principles that guide the growth of snowflakes, the shapes of galaxies, and the creation of every unique human.

I never saw Sarah again. My rotation on the pediatric ward ended that week. I had heard that she required a third surgery because there were complications, but after that I never learned of her fate.

I like to think that maybe she is still watching those beautiful, infinite, multicolored fractals unfolding somewhere, somehow.

The Time Traveler

We humans are born time travelers. No, we don't yet have the ability to physically propel ourselves in strange machines through space-time wormholes and across eons of time past or future. Theoretical physicists assure us that this may indeed be possible someday as the idea does not seem to violate the laws of physics, at least as we understand them today. But for now, however, we must be content with the unique human ability of traveling through imaginary time by way of our precious memories. Animals, both reptiles and mammals, may be frozen in the eternal now. But not us; we can ruminate over our past and imagine our futures. This uniquely human power is both a gift and a curse.

I can mentally time-travel to decades ago and remember with great clarity the joy and excitement of sledding for many hours down the hill behind my grandparents' house. I can also revisit my backyard, where years ago I enjoyed a snowball fight one wintry day with my children.

From an evolutionary point of view, this mental time travel may have been essential for our ancestors' survival. The tree shrews of seventy million years ago had to remember to take cover by day, lest the great dinosaur lizards crush them into oblivion. Our early Neanderthal cousins had to mentally record their daily dangers if they were to have any hope of surviving the travails of hunting, gathering, and tool-making.

Deep in the brain, just above the brain stem and just below the temporal lobes, lays the ancient limbic system. This collection of neural circuitry mediates memory, emotionality, and learning. When I recall the death of a loved one or remember wrestling with my children in their youngest years, it is this part of my brain that allows me to experience these recollections with sadness or joy. All of our memories seem to be stored in the hippocampi, deep in the temporal lobes, one on the right and one on the left, especially our autobiographical memories, and it is in this part of our brain that our cherished stored experiences are infused with joy, sadness, fear, and anger. This is why we just don't recollect a series of sterile cinematic images when we remember—we also relive our experiences.

The past experiences encoded deep in our brain as memories are what make each of us unique individuals. There are myriad events that make up our lives, particularly our childhood, which forge a specific personality for each of us with the help of genetics (nature) but molded by experience (nurture). It is our big brain—our cerebral cortex particularly—that allows us to instantly access remote and recent memories, thereby freeing us from the eternal now that our primate ancestors were locked into. Space and time no longer bind our minds because of our capacity to remember. We take for granted this remarkable ability, at least until it is taken away from us.

Mrs. Dorothy Castiglenio was a seventy-two-year-old Italian immigrant who came to New York at the age of sixteen with her parents and siblings, carrying all her worldly possessions in a small burlap suitcase. She raised a family and was married for over fifty years until the recent death of her husband. She was now living with one of her daughters. Her family physician, at the request of her children, had recommended a neurological consultation for "altered mental status," a generic term that has entered the medical lexicon and describes any person who presents with some troubling change in his or her ability to think, reason, remember, or otherwise behave in a normal fashion. Under this all-encompassing term, a person who is mildly intoxicated from a few glasses of wine or who is in deep coma from a sudden brain hemorrhage is suffering from "altered mental status." The phrase is obviously vague enough to be almost worthless.

Mrs. C. (as I called her) was neither drunk nor in a coma. In fact, she was pleasant, cordial, gracious, and elegant. She was smartly dressed with clear facial features and flowing gray hair. When I engaged her in conversation, the topic turned to recent events. This was when she expressed her sadness over the assassination of President John F. Kennedy. She was very concerned because she wondered who would now run the country, particularly given the state of the Cold War. When I explained to her that she was talking about something that occurred over fifty years ago, she completely disregarded me.

The harsh fluorescent light of my exam room hardened her facial lines. I dimmed the lights so I could examine her pupils and optic nerves with my ophthalmoscope. Oddly, as she bent her head upward to allow me to examine her eyes, she seemed to be smiling at the bright ceiling lamp.

That old adage about the eyes being the windows of the soul was prescient. With enough skill, a learned observer can peer into those black pools and find evidence of brain tumor or stroke. The optic nerves, physical extensions of the brain, can be readily observed. With one eye peering into another, I did not see any problem. But clearly there was a problem. Mrs. C. was confused. She could speak eloquently about the past, her past. Memories about her childhood, her journey from Italy to New York, her father's backyard fig trees, and even political history were all lucidly preserved and recalled. She could not, however, recognize her daughter, identifying her only as "you know, my lady who helps." She could not tell me how she spent her morning or even tell me the names of her children or deceased husband.

I continued with my neurological rituals as her daughter watched anxiously. I seemed to be confirming what she knew all along. Asked to name simple objects, such as a thumb or a button, she would struggle. Mrs. C. did admit frustration over one issue. She could not accurately create any of her longtime, favorite kitchen recipes like lasagna or pasta fagioli. The memory of her recipes was still preserved. She knew ingredients and amounts, but it was the logic of the kitchen that eluded her. Location and purpose of utensils, cups, spoons, baking pans, and stove dials eluded her. Yet Mrs. C. was blissfully, and perhaps mercifully, unaware of most of her plight. She would often repeat to me, "Young fella, you're making a mountain out of a nothing at all. I'm doing just fine." This wasn't the denial of Freudian psychology—the subconscious mind not allowing for recognition of something too emotionally painful to acknowledge—but rather complete unawareness of her incapacities due to damaged brain circuitry (referred to as "anosognosia" in my profession's technical jargon).

I picked up my reflex hammer and continued the formalities of the neurological exam. I dutifully ordered some of the standard diagnostic tests, including a brain MRI and an EEG (electroencephalogram). The first provides us with a series of clear, high-resolution brain images while the second is a recording of the brain's electrical activity. These studies would prove to be relatively normal. It is always humbling to see how some of our most powerful diagnostic tools can reveal so little about what's going on inside the mind of someone obviously suffering from a ravaging disease.

Mrs. C.'s brain was no longer an electrochemical concert seamlessly producing self-awareness and memory. It was becoming a cacophony of fragmented thoughts and jumbled recollections. Dementia, whether it be the most common Alzheimer's type or rarer varieties, slowly robs a person of language, reason, judgment, and perhaps most precious to the individual self, memory. No two humans can have the same set of experiences; therefore, all memories are unique, irreplaceable, and irreproducible. Mrs. C. was gradually becoming trapped in a world of distant, fragmented memories, a prisoner lost in some confused past and unable to travel back to the living present. I put down my reflex hammer and sat back down.

I began my perfunctory discussion of dementia, discussing its natural history of inexorable progression, limited treatment options, and the neuropathology of brain plaques and tangles that damage the hippocampi and amygdalae, the seats of memory and emotion. I've learned over the years, like most in my profession, the occupational hazard of hiding from a patient's tragedy with matter-of-fact scientific discussion. All eyes in the room swelled with tears, except for the victim's. She remained resolute, mercifully dumbstruck.

Several years later she was admitted to a nursing home. Now, at seventy-six, she appeared haggard and silvery. Her thin, frail body sat in a rocking chair. Her room was nicely appointed with photographs of the children and grandchildren; one archival-looking black-and-white photo revealed a young, vibrant Mrs. C. and her husband. At this point she could recognize none of them. I turned on the overhead fluorescent lights as the room was becoming shadowy in the early evening light. She could tell me her name, but even the simplest conversation eluded her, and she certainly had no idea who I was. She fixated on those harsh overhead lamps, much like she did years ago in my exam room. And again, she seemed to faintly smile.

A few months later, one of her daughters called me to let me know that her mother had died quietly in her sleep. The medical staff explained that it was probably a sudden heart attack or blood clot. The family recognized this for what it was—a kind and painless end to an otherwise wretched last few years of life.

I often wonder what the last thoughts would have been for a person like Mrs. C. With her brain scarred by short-circuited dying neurons, her mind might be nothing more than a buzzing chaos of incomprehensible images and splintered thoughts. But deep in her temporal lobes, still glowing like fading embers, some of her oldest and most cherished memories might still be clear and intact. Perhaps when she smiled at those fluorescent ceiling lamps—solar-like in their brightness—she was remembering being a young girl again in her father's garden in Italy, her face warmed by the sunlight filtering through the big green fig leaves in that faraway place so long ago.

Without memory we quickly become strangers in a strange land, lost in a twilight zone of unfamiliar faces, voices, and sights. One's beloved home for decades can become a mysterious landscape filled with fear and even paranoia. Beloved family members—children, siblings, a spouse—can become suspicious doppelgangers, vaguely recognized and mistrusted. This is much of how Mrs. C. spent her last years of life. But imagine a different type of stranded time traveler, one who is trapped in a nightmare of perpetual forgetfulness.

Joe A. is what we called him at a New York City hospital where I interned. The "A" stood for "alcoholic." Picked up off the grimy streets of Hell's Kitchen before the neighborhood became sanitized and gentrified many years ago, he was in his late forties but looked much more weathered and worn before his time ("appears older than stated age" is a standard, nonjudgmental medical phrase I was taught to write in my History and Physical note). He told me his first name but not his last for fear of some unspoken retribution. Although Joe A. had been living on the streets and sometimes in shelters, the rumor was that once upon a time he was a successful banker who lost his wife, children, and career for the solace of drink and heroin—although he maintained that the latter was only a brief vice years ago. He periodically made his way into the ER, often brought in by EMS crews that would find him roaming the neighborhood or bedding down, semiconscious, in one of the shadowy hospital alleys. One night the obligations of my call schedule stationed me in the emergency room, and it was my turn to encounter him.

Drenched with the odor of the street and alcohol, wearing blue jeans and a tattered monogrammed Ralph Lauren shirt (initials BGV on the pocket), he was obviously intoxicated. My role as an intern was to examine him and to make certain that there was no immediate life-threatening medical or neurological issue that needed to be addressed, as alcoholics can often suffer serious head trauma, meningitis, endocarditis, and a large array of other medical conditions that I had only read about in textbooks until now.

"Hi, Joe. I'm Dr. Adamo, the ER intern on call tonight. I don't think we've met before. How are you doing?" I asked. "Is your name really Joe?"

With his blue eyes and salt-and-pepper hair, he looked somewhat patrician. He answered, "You can call me Joe." He gave a quick glance at me and his shirt monogram, and as if to read my mind, he added, "Those initials are mine…but these days I just go by 'Joe'."

I went about my intern ritual. I drew blood for basic labs—electrolytes, liver and kidney function, and blood count. I listened to his heart and breath sounds, tapped on his limbs with my reflex hammer, and, just a little curious about a patient whom all the interns knew of, started to talk to him.

I began my basic mental status protocol. He was alert and fully oriented despite being mildly inebriated. It was an autumn night, and he must have been cold outside. He asked for another blanket. His presidential recall was excellent all the way back to Eisenhower—an unusual feat for most people in better circumstances. He wasn't delusional or psychotic. In fact his demeanor was somber. He was fairly articulate—not what you'd usually expect from a homeless man, or at least not typically what I was used to dealing with. Psychotic bag ladies, HIV-infected junkies, and vagabond psychiatric patients were the more usual midnight denizens of this emergency room.

With my basic intern duties completed, and having ruled

out that my patient was suffering any immediate life-threatening disorder, I decided to talk to him for a little while. After all, he was kind of an ER legend at the time for reasons I hadn't yet realized.

"How long have you been homeless, Joe?" I asked with professional aloofness, the kind that I learned early in a big city hospital where you try to ignore, or pretend to ignore, tragedy.

"I've kind of lost track, you know; it's been many years now." He seemed eager to talk. Very few people ever asked him personal questions, and I think he seemed pleased that someone was taking an interest in him that wasn't purely medical.

"It wasn't always like this. I had a family—a wife and two kids—a big house in Westchester. I was successful, traded on Wall Street. I started drinking a lot, cocaine too. It made me bipolar. Everything fell apart."

I was silent and perhaps a little stunned. He went on with his midnight confession.

"I haven't seen my kids in over a decade. I'm ashamed. I don't even think they know I'm alive." His voice quivered, but he remained resolute.

I was silent. It finally dawned on me that he once had a life, an enviable life, but now he lived on the streets, often drunk and filthy.

My beeper went off, and I was paged to draw a blood sugar level on an in-patient on one of the wards. I excused myself and told Joe I would be back soon. I was gone for about half an hour or so. I returned to see my ER patient still lying on his gurney. He looked at me vacantly. I started to discuss the medical treatment I had planned for him: alcohol detox regimen, IV fluids and vitamins, social service consult, etc. It became obvious that he had no recollection of who I was. In fact, he was rather suspicious of me, insisting that I was some "hospital investigator" who was looking into a money-laundering scam that may have involved him. I went through the differential diagnoses of possible causes of this behavior: acute psychosis, schizophrenia, acute cocaine toxicity, and delirium tremens, but none of them fit. He was rational a few minutes ago. Now he was paranoid but still very much coherent.

He wasn't tremulous or agitated, so I knew this wasn't acute alcohol withdrawal or the "DTs." He clearly did not recall the fact that we had just talked, nor did he recollect the fact that I performed an entire medical examination on him. I wasn't even sure that he recognized me. He tried to convince me that we recently had a meeting, but its purpose was to discuss his lost investments. He was confabulating—making up stories to fill in his memory gaps. The mind desperately tries to maintain a coherent narrative, even at the expense of reality. Joe could not retain recent memories, immediate recall. He was stuck in an eternal now, haunted by distant intact memories of his former life.

The attending neurologist was called for a consult. I remember he was tall and bearded, very erudite looking. Perhaps he was one of my first living inspirations to pursue neurology. He said, somewhat arrogantly, that the diagnosis was obvious. "Wernicke-Korsakoff's encephalopathy, you will see this a lot at a city hospital like this one," he announced. "These folks damage their temporal lobes, hippocampi, mammillary bodies—you know, those areas of the brain that seem most susceptible to the toxic effects of alcohol. Some of this may be reversible. We'll start him on intravenous thiamine which should help; it's helped in the past. Remote memories, years and decades ago, can be well preserved, but recent stuff is lost almost immediately."

He was right. Thiamine (and other B-vitamins) is deficient in alcoholics. The supplementation quickly helped, and in a couple of days he was apologetic about his memory lapses. The other interns and I talked about helping him reconnect with his children. We were all moved by his story, whose accuracy had apparently been at least partially corroborated. As the days passed, he became more irritable and anxious despite treatment with Valium to reduce these alcohol withdrawal symptoms. One late night, unknown to the covering resident and nursing staff, he pulled the IV line from his arm, got dressed, and walked out of the hospital. Maybe he was desperate for a drink. Maybe he couldn't bear the thought of seeing his children after all these years. Maybe he was just ashamed of himself as he once told me.

The benefit of the thiamine vitamin therapy would wane quickly. He would soon be trapped back again in a twilight zone of perpetual forgetfulness. Perhaps that's how he wanted it. He could remember only that stately suburban house in the bright daylight and his wife sitting on the porch steps, watching him play with his children on the lawn. He could stay there forever.

Reptilian Housewives

THE HUMAN FACE—IT can convey a seemingly infinite array of expressions, emotions, even ideas. It wasn't always this way. It took a few hundred million years of evolution to develop the neurological architecture to achieve this. Look at some our most remote ancestors. Dinosaurs have the blank, expressionless visage of all reptiles. Fish, sea slugs, and worms can convey no meaning with their empty eyes. Even the tree shrews and lemurs, our first primate ancestors, have nothing more than a wide-eyed stare. The chimpanzees, for all the DNA we share with them, have a limited facial repertoire. No, it is just the human who cannot only convey all of the primary emotions with such vividness—happiness, sadness, anger, fear, disgust—but also all of the vast subtleties—jealousy, flirtation, distrust, interest, reluctance, cynicism, love. Charles Darwin recognized this and realized the role of human evolution in producing this wonderful gift. Some facial expressions, such as the gaping-eye stare of fear or the wide-mouthed smile of joy, may be universal and innate. Others, like the snarl of jealousy, may be learned or cultural. But it is the ability of facial expressions to convey so much nonverbal information that is uniquely human.

There are several unfortunate neurological conditions that can forever alter a person's ability to convey obvious feelings with emotion. Stroke victims often have facial weakness as do muscular dystrophy patients. Bell's palsy patients develop temporary facial droops, which they find incredibly frustrating. It's hard to imagine how anyone would want to deliberately induce facial weakness and paralysis, but it has become a multibillion-dollar cosmetic industry in America. It's called Botox.

Botox is the commercial name for botulinum toxin, which is secreted by the same bacteria that causes the dreaded but fortunately now rare infection botulism. It can be lethal because it causes paralysis of skeletal muscles like the facial muscles. The dreaded paralysis can be beneficial if you're looking to stop those inevitable fine wrinkles around the eyes, mouth, and forehead. The problem is that those exquisite muscles, the product of millions of years of evolution, are crucial to conveying the daily emotions that we take for granted in our facial expressions. Without free use of those facial muscles, our expressions can become as superficial as the emoticons we use in e-mailing and texting.

Sandra M. was an attractive housewife in her early forties. Her two children had already started college. She was, as far as I knew, happily married and enjoyed a stable and affluent life in suburbia. She had been treated for mild depression in the past but was otherwise healthy. Although physically attractive and youthful, somewhere along the way she became convinced that she needed to try to recapture her once radiant twenty-five-year-old face. In a society obsessed with the fanatical pursuit of youth, where mothers try to emulate their teenage daughters' demeanors and lifestyles—and where advancing age is seen, perversely, as a fate worse than death—this did not seem surprising.

Botox injections have become widely available in general medical and dermatologists' offices throughout the country. Plastic surgeons, thanks in part to Botox availability, now enjoy prominence not only in wealthy neighborhoods but in working class ones as well. The fountain of youth, or at least its illusion, is but a scalpel's cut or needle's injection away.

Sandra had come to see me for a neurological consultation regarding the possibility of Botox injections. As a neurologist I do not provide such treatment for merely cosmetic reasons (although neurologists these days do treat certain conditions with Botox injections, such as dystonia and migraine). Sandra was advised to see me in order to get some advice regarding potential complications of this widely used therapy. We discussed some well-known adverse effects like temporary and prolonged paralysis of some of the facial muscles, as well as rarer but more serious complications such as difficulty breathing and swallowing. I was struck by her bright face, full of expression, that still suggested youthfulness. I thought that it was rather odd that she was even considering these treatments, and so I asked further about possible depression or anxiety, but she showed no trace of this. By all accounts, this was a normal, well-adjusted woman who simply wanted to "look my best." And what was wrong with this? After all, isn't the adage of every celebrity TV show and self-help guru to "look and be the best you can" and "realize your full potential," which in our society, governed by increasing superficiality, really means to look as young as you possibly can—even if it requires invasive medical intervention, being needled and prodded, or having flesh ripped and toxins pumped into your body. Damn the soul; it's the body that the world wants. I wished her good luck in her pursuit, and she left my office ready to follow her wishes.

The obsession with youth has never been as pervasive as it is today. We have been called a culture of narcissism. The fixation with the body and its appearance has become so intense it mimics the pathological extremes that we see in young anorexics and bulimics, who binge and purge until they become skeletal. The victims of these disorders can't even imagine that they're not obese. We mechanically suck the fat out of the overweight, tie knots around stomachs to shrink them, surgically tighten the face musculature so it's so taught a simple smile might unravel a visage, and even peroxide bleach cigarette-stained teeth—all this to create the illusion of health. We buy bogus vitamin supplements or eagerly wait for the next even more dangerous diet fad in the hopes that it will bring newfound self-fulfillment.

And so Sandra saw her plastic surgeon, paid with her Visa card, and waited to be beautiful again.

She returned unexpectedly to my office a few months later. She had already received several Botox facial injections. She was ambivalent about the results but wanted to continue. She explained that she was concerned about the lack of facial movement. Blinking, wrinkling the forehead, even a wide smile had all become difficult. I explained that this was inevitable given that the very purpose of the botulinum toxin is to work as a paralyzing agent. This is in fact why the Clostridium botulinum bacteria can cause such a lethal infection. The Botox injections were deliberately weakening her muscles, as less movement in the facial muscles meant less wrinkling. As I spoke with her, I could not help but recall the all too common TV images of female (and male) news reporters and talk show celebrities who recite tragic stories and sports updates with the same blank, wide-eyed gaze, their faces paralyzed and preserved with that elixir of youth. I warned her about proceeding although there was no legitimate neurological reason that I could give her. Botox is widely considered safe and effective for its intended cosmetic purpose and is FDA approved.

A month later I received a phone call from her husband who had been conspicuously absent during Sandra's previous visits to my office. He was concerned about what he believed was a fixation or obsession with her Botox injections. He suspected that she was seeing more than one plastic surgeon for her injections and that she was lying about this to her doctors. He even speculated that perhaps she was somehow self-injecting with Botox between visits to the plastic surgeons. She was using various codeine painkillers as well to ease the soreness from the multiple needle sticks. He explained that her face was becoming more bloated and blank and that, somehow, as if to mimic her physical appearance, she too was becoming more detached and aloof. Intimacy had all but stopped, and she was becoming reclusive. I recommended that he discuss these concerns immediately with her plastic surgeon and arrange for a psychiatric consultation. I could hear the worry in his voice.

Reptiles don't have an amygdala or neocortex. It took many millions of eons after the dinosaur age for the primates to evolve these advanced brain structures that allow us to appreciate and react to all the nuances of emotion and not just fear, that most primordial of all emotions. It is only the human brain that can grasp all the subtle meanings expressed in a smile, frown, wink, or snarl. It is only the human face that has the exquisite musculature to produce all the subtle variations of a simple smile, frown, wink, or snarl. Even our ancient primate ancestors, the tree shrews that hid in the dark of night while the great lizards ruled the earth a hundred million years ago, possess only a gaping stare. Gnawing on insects in the dark, they only knew one emotion: fear. It is hard to imagine why we would want to revert back to that cold reptilian gaze, barely able to smile or cry.

With skin surgically taut, Botoxed, and siliconed, we are losing one of the hallmarks of human evolution: the ability to express our emotions and opinions with a simple fold of the brow or hint of a smile. Our faces are becoming much like those empty emoticons, devoid of any real feeling. It is the face of the sociopath.

One night Sandra overdosed on Percocet and Valium, and her husband found her unconscious in one of the upstairs bathrooms. She died an hour later of cardiac respiratory arrest at the local hospital. He explained tearfully, at the funeral, that her once beautiful face was bloated and frozen from all the self-injections. He hoped she was now at peace, but her final facial expression could not reveal that. It would take several months after she was lowered into the ground for the botulinum toxin to wear off and her facial muscles to finally relax. No one would ever gaze upon her final countenance.

Cassandra's Nightmare

If you could know how and when you would die, would you want to? Could you make sensible use of such knowledge? Or would it torment you knowing the how, when, and why you would meet your demise? For some, this is no longer a theoretical consideration but a real-life dilemma. Predictive genetic testing of one's DNA—the molecular blueprint that encodes much of our physical and mental traits—is now becoming increasingly available. Looking into the nucleotide sequence of our DNA can be, for some, like peering into the future. But proceed warily; you may not like what you find.

In Greek mythology there is the famous tale of Cassandra; beautiful and brilliant with dark hair and brooding eyes, she was considered insane. The daughter of a king and queen, she was cursed by Apollo when she rejected his romantic advances. Her curse: she was given the gift of prophecy, but no one would ever believe her accurate predictions of doom and tragedy. This would prove an endless source of frustration and torment for her, as everyone including her own family considered her a liar and a lunatic. She foresaw the demise of her mother Hecuba, the exile of Odysseus, and the fall of Troy; however, she was unable to prevent any of these tragedies because no one believed her predictions. She even knew of her inevitable murder but could do nothing to alter her destiny.

Sarah H. was thirty-eight years old, mother of two young children, and devoted wife. She was raised mainly by her mother and maternal grandparents in rural Pennsylvania. Her father died when she was only a child, and she had only dim recollections of him. The details were murky. He had been a foreman for a local construction company and a family man. While still in his early thirties, his behavior became increasingly unstable and bizarre. He lost his job, became disgruntled with his life, and was ultimately institutionalized with a diagnosis of paranoid schizophrenia. On one visiting day, Sarah's mother found him hanging over a ceiling beam with his trouser belt in a bathroom of the nursing home.

That's when talk about something bad in the family blood started. She remembered hushed family conversations about a curse of madness. The family doctor put forth a diagnosis of "suicide resulting from psychosis of schizophrenia," but that never seemed to make much sense in a man who seemed reasonable up until the last year of his life. Sarah recalled him as a loving father who doted on her mom. A weird combination of sadness and shame silenced any future discussion over his death, or life for that matter, and her father was rarely spoken about again.

Decades later, she appeared in my office with questions.

"I don't really have a neurological problem, or at least not yet as far as I can tell," she explained. "I just need some advice."

This was somewhat unusual. Most patients in the day-to-day grind of a neurology practice present with very specific concerns or symptoms—headache, dizziness, numbness. Sarah was seemingly healthy with none of these.

"I know there are lots of conditions, disease that can now be screened for with genetic testing. I'd like to look into this. I have a family, two young children, a husband." She sounded resolute.

"Well, we just can't screen randomly for diseases. First, we don't really have that kind of medical technology yet, and second, there are only a few specific inheritable diseases that might be worth looking into. It's rather complicated because having a gene and developing the disease that the gene carries are often not directly correlated," I explained. "Some conditions, such as the BRCA gene for breast cancer and the Tay-Sachs screen, can be very predictive, but more often than not the situation is not that simple."

She didn't like my answer. I was being obtuse. She wanted something, I didn't know what, and I was clearly not complying with her.

The Victorian house was cavernous, or at least seemed that way to an eight-year-old child. Playing hide-and-seek could take hours, especially if one was brave enough to take cover in the attic, dark and dusty with a century of memories from her German immigrant grandparents, coal-mining uncles, and a great aunt who sang in the traveling circus. But Sarah knew the house, her childhood home since birth, well enough to usually be the last found. One summer afternoon, her aunt called out to the children to come downstairs. There were unfamiliar cars parked out front, Sarah remembered, and her mom stood silently in the kitchen, where everyone was gathering. It was there that she was told of her father's sudden death, an accident of some kind. She would not learn until years later that it was a suicide, although she recalled the word whispered many times; she even looked it up in the school's Webster's months later. She recalled her mother sobbing and the scent of the fresh pickles, recently sealed in Mason jars, resting on the big wood table.

"My mother won't ever talk about it after all these years, but I do have some recollections. I remember he was a fun dad, and he got along well with everyone. And then suddenly, it seemed, he was in and out of hospitals, although now I know it was really a psychiatric asylum that kind of doubled as a nursing home. We lived in a pretty rural area, and our family doctor still delivered an occasional baby." Sarah was tearful now. "I just want to know what happened and if it's something that can affect my children one day."

She presented to me a thick folder full of frayed, graying

medical records like some ancient archive. She had managed to retrieve them from the psychiatric hospital where her father spent his last days. There were mainly psychiatrist notes. Often schizophrenia was raised as a possible diagnosis. ECT (electroconvulsive therapy) was tried more than once. Still used to this day, the procedure involves literally shocking the brain with electricity while the patient is sedated. It will induce a seizure, and sometimes it may alleviate depression or psychosis in a patient who is not responding to standard medications. There was talk about performing a frontal lobotomy. Long abandoned as barbaric and dangerous, this was once a fairly popular procedure for treating all manner of neurological disorders, including epilepsy, dementia, schizophrenia, and depression. It left its victims in a zombie-like state, severely brain damaged. These medical notes were from the early 1970s, and the procedure was still considered of some benefit in difficult-to-treat cases. I tried desperately to find a neurology consult among all the psychiatric and nursing handwritten notes (no electronic medical records in those days) but with no success. The final official entry, before the death pronouncement, was a simple progress note: patient stable, appears alert and oriented. Resting comfortably.

It is often said that the practice of medicine, neurology in particular, is like detective work. One needs to piece together seemingly disparate signs and symptoms to reach a unifying diagnosis. The entire intellectual process often reminds me of the old TV detective show *Columbo*. Each episode would start with a clear depiction of exactly how the crime, typically a murder, was carried out. The rest of the hour or so illustrated how the brilliant but humble Lieutenant Columbo would figure out how and why the crime was committed and by whom. It's kind of the same reverse engineering we deal with in medicine. Here's the person and their problem. Now tell me, Doctor, how did we get to this and what caused all this? And what can we do about it?

In this case, however, I didn't even have a living patient. Just a tearful daughter and a folder full of dusty records.

There are many neurological diseases where genes and heredity play a strong role. In fact most maladies that afflict humans, from diabetes to cancer, have some genetic influences. Here was a story of a young man who tragically went insane with no explanation. There were, however, some clues to be found in the dank and dusty archived medical notes. A few references to "twitchy arms" or "facial tics" were found in the daily progress notes. There is a condition, rare but well known…

"I've read about lots of these diseases," Sarah announced, unaware of how knowledgeable she had become. "There's multiple sclerosis, muscular dystrophies, heavy metal poisoning, but none of these apply. But there is one—"

And at that point I interrupted her. "You're wondering about Huntington's disease, aren't you?"

"Yes, exactly," she responded somberly.

The condition in question, Huntington's disease, is the quintessential, fatal neurogenetic disorder. It is inexorably progressive and universally results in death, often within just a few years after it is diagnosed. There is no cure or effective treatment at present. The physical and mental breakdown occurs usually in a person's prime, their thirties or forties. It begins insidiously, perhaps with minor personality changes, depression or anxiety symptoms. Incoordination with choreiform (rapid, sudden, jerky involuntary limb or facial movements that can be confused with nervous tics) may ensue. Gradually, its victims become demented, unable to reason, talk rationally or think coherently, and enter a stage of total debilitation, often bed stricken like an elderly person struck with Alzheimer's. Every child of a parent with HD has a 50 percent chance of developing the disease. But it's not as straightforward as that.

The abnormal gene, located on chromosome number 4, has multiple variations. If the rogue DNA sequence repeats more than forty times, the disease will develop in the affected person. If the sequence is less than thirty-six, the person is safe from the dreaded fate. But between thirty-six and forty, there is the possibility—but not inevitability—of Huntington's developing. And even if you carry less than the prerequisite thirty-six, you may still pass on a fatal mutation to one of your children. It would seem that Cassandra can really open up a Pandora's box here.

All this posed a real-life dilemma for Sarah, as does genetic testing for more and more people today. There is no practical benefit to be gained by learning which genetic category one possesses with regard to HD, as no treatment can yet be offered. But knowing your ultimate fate, the approximate likelihood of the how and when, and if your children may be destined for a similar demise may or may not be worth knowing. She agonized over this for weeks.

She called me many times over the ensuing weeks, developing a kind of mental calculus of all possible outcomes if she were to undergo genetic counseling.

"Okay, here's what I've come up with." I could hear the exasperation in her voice. "If I learn that I don't carry the gene, that will be great knowledge. If I learn that I do carry it, then I can at least prepare somehow. But maybe it would be better not to know since there's nothing I could do about it anyway. I might live in fear if I did know, just waiting for any sign of the disease. I don't know…and what if the results are indeterminate? Then I'm back where I started."

I empathized and explained, "Sarah, this is a door only you can open or close."

After months of procrastination, discussion with her husband, and second and third opinions, she finally resolved to undergo genetic counseling at a university hospital. She had the blood tests and waited weeks before allowing the geneticist to divulge the results to her.

"The trinucleotide repeat count on the HTT gene is thirty-eight. Smack right in the damn middle of indeterminate. Maybe fifty-fifty chance for me and my kids of developing some form of the disease." There seemed to be some relief in her voice.

"The results could have been much worse," I responded reassuringly.

She nodded in agreement. "Still, not knowing one way or the other…," she quickly replied.

I looked at her and smiled. "That's probably the best that most of us can ever hope for."

Do Helicopters Eat Their Young?

The mind constructs, or represents, the reality outside of our heads using our senses: wavelengths of light, tremors of air; it fills in the gaps that our senses don't provide using imagination. Such is the nature of its vast information-processing ability that sometimes the mind can only create a crude representation of the world like Plato's cave dwellers, who only catch glimpses of flickering shadows on the wall and not the true reality that they reflect. Nonetheless, our brains do a pretty good job of identifying everything that's out there. We have created science with its power to comprehend nature and make accurate observations and predictions about the universe around us. And we have art, which allows the mind's eye to turn inward in order to understand our humanity. Sometimes, however, the brain gets things terribly wrong. Synapses cross-fire, leagues of neurons misbehave, and chemical neurotransmitters like dopamine flood the brain. The results are often tragically disabling.

The mind can construct its own perverse shadow world, which bears little resemblance to reality. Some can struggle against such disease with every fiber of their being; many must succumb to it and live in a state of dependency, often spending their lives in and out of institutions.

Hell's Kitchen, late 1980s, summertime. I was a young intern in the big city. Not yet married with children, I was naive in ways I couldn't imagine but filled with the kind of knowledge that comes out of heavy textbooks. The kind of books I lugged around for a decade and pored over for countless hours and days learning anatomy, neurophysiology, and neuropathology in the hopes of knowing, or hoping to know, how to deal with real, live patients.

Homelessness was a major problem in Manhattan during that decade, particularly because of the epidemic of psychiatric in-patient facilities closing. The chronic mentally ill were released by the thousands with the promise of outpatient care. Many of them were without families or homes, and as a result they ended up on the streets living out of shopping carts along sidewalks, underpasses, and in the labyrinths of the dirty subway system. I met one of the homeless victims on a hot July afternoon.

"Little Bob" was escorted to the emergency room by a couple of police officers. He was acting belligerent—cursing at the hazy sky—when some local store owners called the police. His behavior was frightening some of the youthful upscale patrons of a newly minted row of restaurants that had recently cropped up in the neighborhood, an early sign of that new sociological phenomenon now known as gentrification. The moniker "Little Bob" was apparently given to him by the locals with a sense of irony, as he was about six foot five with a heavy frame. His real name was unknown.

Unkempt, grimy with sweat, and wearing blue jeans and a "Blondie" T-shirt, we determined that he was dehydrated and mildly hyperthermic. We started a round of IV fluids, thiamine, and multivitamins. We talked about Wernicke's encephalopathy and Korsakoff's syndrome, both commonly seen in alcoholics, which we assumed he was. He had to be hosed down with antiseptic soap in the ER showering stall to wash away the city dirt and lice. He downed two hospital cheeseburgers, which we promised him as a reward if he would finally agree to undergo a brain CT, which he did. We wanted to make sure we didn't miss a traumatic head injury like a subdural hematoma, not unusual among the homeless, particularly alcoholics. Up until now, he spoke little other than to answer some basic medical questions and to say his name was Bob.

"Tell us your name," we began our formal mental status exam.

"Bob, just Bob, that's all I'm saying for now," he curtly responded.

He knew who the president was (Reagan). He knew the month, day, and year. He seemed coherent but reticent about discussing any personal history. Nonetheless, his language was sensible, not aphasic. He understood he was in a hospital. But he wasn't quite right. Somber, with a blank stare, he intermittently swatted away at gnats that didn't seem to be there.

His labs came back and looked rather normal, despite some obvious dehydration. Urine toxicology showed no evidence of illicit drugs, such as cocaine or amphetamines, and no trace of narcotics. The brain CT was normal as well. We talked about the possibility of doing a spinal tap, but there were really no signs of meningitis, such as fever or elevated white blood cell count. His behavior was a little odd, but he wasn't delirious or confused by any means. He was transferred from the ER to a regular bed on the medical floor with the admission diagnosis of dehydration—a diagnosis that basically gave us medical justification for admitting him while we could look into why exactly this young man, probably around my age at the time, was aimlessly roaming the west side of Manhattan.

Being the lowly intern, I was assigned to try to extract a complete history from Little Bob. I introduced myself, sat on a chair at his bedside, and got to it.

After taking care of the perfunctory details like past medical history, of which there was nothing significant, at least from what he would divulge to me, I began my neurological mental status exam. He was calm and coherent and fully oriented to person, place, time, and circumstance as we routinely describe patients. He seemed to have a pretty good fund of knowledge. He knew about the big news story of the year—President Reagan and the Iran-Contra arms affair. He was clearly intelligent and articulate.

"How long have you been on the street? Where were you living before?" I asked.

"Well, I have a nice home and two parents who live on the Upper East Side, but I had to leave. There were troubles, things I couldn't reckon with the sphere of this mundane existence. It's like '*Soylent Green* is people,' you know what I mean?"

I recognized the science-fiction movie reference—Charlton Heston's famous line in the dystopian future when his character discovers that the green wafers being fed to the starving masses are made of recycled dead humans.

He went on, seemingly invigorated by his revelation. "It's as if even the very atoms that make up this city are toxic and there's no way to get things back. It's embedded in the mind matter, and it's full of tachyons. And no, it's not the hand of God…this is bigger than that. You can't even imagine. I've been roaming the streets trying to get a handle on this." His eyes twitched.

"Have you ever been treated for any psychiatric disorders?" I asked bluntly.

"I'm okay, and I don't use drugs," he responded, avoiding my question.

"Okay," I quickly said. Then I pushed for him to explain further, fascinated by his ramblings.

"Look, I spent a year at Princeton University. I was gonna be a physics major. Mathematics is the language of science, and I wanted to work on cosmology, you know, the Big Bang and all. But I was getting sick at the atomic level. They told me this would happen. They told me all along!" He started to look nervous, and his speech got more pressured as if he were trying to rid himself of each toxic atom by spewing as many words as he could.

At this point I was a little perplexed. Yes, I knew there was something wrong here, but it wasn't clear to me how wrong. Despite his weirdness, he was articulate and seemed to have something important he was trying to get out, almost against his mind's will.

The social worker had done some research. We found out his real name was Robert Dercer. He had been admitted to the hospital previously for a minor injury. It appeared that he was living with his parents uptown like he said. His father was a well-known real estate broker in the city. He was a rich kid, and he really did go to Princeton for about a year.

The next morning, before reporting for official rounds with my chief resident and attending, I checked in on Robert. He was eating breakfast, a typical hospital tray of pancakes, oatmeal, and a slice of ham, all of which he seemed to savor. Lying alongside of the bed was a string of sheets, four or five, tied together making one long twisted rope. It looked like a noose was fashioned at the end. I asked him what this was.

"You know, if things get bad. It's like the cyanide capsules they give to secret agents if they're captured by the enemy." He smiled widely, as if to mock my own worried expression.

I called a stat psychiatry consult.

White-haired and disheveled, like a harried college professor, Dr. Dreuf came by quickly after the consult was called. Suicidal ideation, suicidal attempts, violence, and acute psychosis are basically the few psychiatric emergencies that exist. The first thing the doctor did was to call in an order for a "one-to-one observation," meaning a nurse or staff member would always be at the patient's bedside to make certain he couldn't successfully carry out his threatened suicide attempts.

Dr. D., the familiar name by which we often referred to him, sat at the bedside. He was tall and heavy set and could be little intimidating before you got to know him. Bob sat up and pushed his finished breakfast tray over.

"You know why they called me to see you, Bob?" he asked sternly.

"Yes, they think I might hurt myself…but I was just taking precautions, you know," he answered meekly.

The psychiatric interview is supposed to be carried out in a very specific format. You start by assessing the patient's physical appearance, mood, and affect. Later on you analyze their judgment, insight, and general cognition. Finally, you classify your various diagnoses into different axes based on the *Diagnostic and Statistical Manual of Mental Disorders* (DMS), the bible of up-to-date psychiatric classification. Dr. D., however, took a more conversational approach. I remember thinking, like many things in life, once you gain real-world experience, you can dispense with the by-the-numbers cookbook and become a chef, improvising as you move along.

About halfway into the interview, it started to become very evident that our patient wasn't just quirky. There was something seriously wrong with him.

"Things started going badly after my first semester at Princeton. I mean I had good grades, but it was a struggle. I knew I was getting sick. The atomic poisons where seeping into me. I knew this was kind of crazy, but I couldn't get it out of my mind. You know in quantum mechanics there's this idea of parallel universes, an infinite number of them where all possible permutations of every event can occur. I started to reason that somehow there was a crossover like a tear in the space-time framework that resulted in this disease traveling. And then the voices started. At first it was just whispers, but then it would wake me up at night."

"Did these voices tell you to hurt yourself or anyone else?" Dr. D. politely asked.

"No, but they told me I was getting sick…and maybe that the university was involved, deliberately causing this so I couldn't uncover the whole mind-matter mystery thing."

We later learned that Bob had been in and out of hospitals for medical evaluations regarding various symptoms—headaches, fatigue, nausea. His workups were always normal. I knew enough psychiatry to realize that our patient was psychotic, what seemed real to him wasn't. He had paranoid delusions, was seeing or hearing things that weren't real, and had become increasing withdrawn and socially isolated to the point that he preferred living on the streets of Manhattan rather than in his comfortable upscale condo with his family.

"Dr. Adamo, is there anything else you'd like to ask our patient?" For some reason Dr. D. singled me out in the room with two other residents and a medical student.

I didn't want to ask him anything. Getting to know more about his life, I started to realize what a sad tragedy it was. He was my age and his life was unraveling. I didn't think I had the right to ask him anything after listening to this.

My mind raced to come up with something, something that wouldn't be too personal. I felt that I might humiliate him if I forced him to reveal more bizarre details about his condition. He was obviously highly intelligent, and I felt he shouldn't have to suffer more indignity. So I asked him something as benign and impersonal as I could come up with, given the circumstances.

"Robert, do helicopters eat their young?" I blurted out.

I had read about this kind of iconic question in psychiatry in my pocket handbook, the kind that interns stuff inside their white lab coats, although these days they have been replaced by iPhone medical apps and tablets that allow for instantaneous research on any such subject. It's kind of a trick question. A normal, rational person will instantly recognize this. Helicopters are not living creatures. They don't produce young and certainly can't eat them in any event. A person who is cognitively impaired from dementia or has disorganized psychotic thought patterns may not recognize this and will try to rationalize the question or explain it with an answer.

He gave me a quizzical look and paused before answering. "I'm not sure what you are trying to imply. Of course the implication is that biological organisms can eat their young if they are so inclined. Helicopters can be vulnerable, you know, but I'm not sure what the intent would be from a survival standpoint. I guess the mothers can…but not typically the fathers," he finally concluded with a puzzled look.

We were silent, trying to process his murky answer.

Dr. D. invited us into the conference room. "Any ideas?" he asked and scanned the room. We dutifully went through the differential diagnoses, organic etiologies first: hepatic encephalopathy, temporal lobe tumor, drug-induced delirium, heavy metal toxicity. None of them fit the clinical picture. Labs and scans were all normal, and there was no evidence that he abused alcohol. No, we all concluded, this had to be psychiatric.

The psychiatrist said, "It's definitely a type of schizophrenia with paranoid features. His brain is a firestorm of neurotransmitters—dopamine, serotonin, norepinephrine—out of control. We'll start haloperidol. Hopefully, that will help with the paranoid delusions and auditory hallucinations. He's a very bright kid. It's a damn shame. Theoretical physics would have been a perfect profession for him, requires no social interaction. You can be a complete loner, alone with your thoughts and a chalkboard of equations. We'll see how he does."

Looking back, I can't help but think of John Nash, the

Nobel Prize-winning economist who suffered from paranoid schizophrenia as well (subject of the movie biopic *A Beautiful Mind*). But as far as I know, my patient never achieved that kind of professional success. He was eventually discharged to his home with his parents on a regimen of several neuroleptic drugs, including the classic haloperidol, a dopamine antagonist which reduces the activity of that neurotransmitter in the cerebral cortex and limbic system.

About six months later, while in the emergency room admitting an elderly stroke patient, I heard a familiar voice in the next cubicle. It was Bob. He recognized me instantly and smiled.

"Got into a little scuffle," he said, pointing to a laceration on his knee that was being sutured. He was still obviously having issues, but he seemed more clear-eyed and astute.

"They're going to let me enroll in some physics courses at City (college). We'll see how that goes."

I smiled and nodded approvingly.

"And by the way"—he smiled back—"I figured out the answer to your helicopter question…only if they're really hungry!"

I laughed out loud and started my walk down the corridor.

The Eternal Vigil

Consciousness is the fire of the mind. It might very well be the ultimate purpose of life and the universe. Death may be nothing less than the permanent extinction of this magical self-awareness. Every joy and tragedy in life is predicated on it, yet its origin and purpose remain a complete mystery.

The consult was called in as a second opinion. I mumbled under my breath when I read the note my secretary left on my desk. Second-opinion consults are the orphans of neurology consults. It can often be a gratuitous exercise in futility. There are typically three categories of this species. The first is possible malpractice. The family, a spouse for instance, is requesting a second neurologist to review a case because they believe the first neurologist screwed up (which may or may not be the case). The second type is spurred by the belief that all the previous doctors caring for the patient may not have considered a possible beneficial treatment. This is rarely the case, but it is sometimes a legitimate concern and sometimes just desperate grasping at straws. Finally, there is the third category: the family is requesting a second opinion because they simply don't like the original neurologist. Perhaps they view him or her as arrogant, obnoxious, or incompetent, and they have lost confidence in anything he or she says or does.

This second opinion fell into none of the above categories.

The hurried teenage girl was driving her blue VW Beetle onto the main highway from the entrance ramp. Distracted by her text messaging, she didn't notice the construction up ahead, nor was she aware of the working crew, the orange traffic cones, or the highway vehicles. She accelerated quickly to merge into the traffic and plowed into the construction zone, hitting one of the men head on at about fifty miles per hour.

"That was over two years ago, Doctor. They rushed him to the hospital, unconscious. He had brain surgery to drain the blood out, but he never woke up. He's been in a nursing home since then. His wife remarried and his teenage children visit less often than they used to. It must be hard to see him like that. But I visit every day. I haven't missed a day in a year and a half. How can I? I'm his mother…that's what I'm supposed to do."

"What kind of state is your son…?" I hesitated not knowing his name.

"Joe, his name is Joe, Doctor."

"What kind of condition is Joe in? Can he talk at all, breath on his own, walk?"

"They say it's PVS, you know."

"Yes, of course."

"I'm sure you've seen cases like this. Major traumatic brain injury. But he never woke up. He just lays there, stares. Doesn't move. Has a feeding tube. Never says a word, but I think maybe he knows when I'm there. It's as if he's waiting for something."

She spoke slowly, deliberately, as if she had said these words so many times before that they no longer had the emotional impact they once had. Or maybe she was just trying to sound that way—professional and detached like the countless doctors she had spoken to over the past many months.

"I wonder if he's getting a little better. I just want a good neurologist to take a look at him. I know sometimes people with so-called irreversible brain damage do get better. The nursing home doctors say that's impossible and I just have to accept his fate, and I understand that but…sometimes I just wonder…maybe my son is still there…inside that rotting body being pumped with synthetic sludge."

I agreed to see her son at the nursing home.

Persistent vegetative state or PVS: the phrase almost became a household word with the case of Terry Schiavo, the lady in an irreversible coma after suffering cardiac arrest. Her story gripped the nation as the family struggled with whether or not to discontinue her feeding tube (ultimately it was disconnected and she mercifully died in 2005). The victims typically suffer some kind of catastrophic event—a stroke, cardiac arrest, or in this case, massive head trauma. After the turmoil of brain surgery, ICU care, breathing machines, and countless doctors and nurses, a nightmarish scenario starts to emerge. The victim appears awake; he or she may even have normal sleep/wake cycles. They sit in bed, rarely show any movement, and stare blankly, although they may sometimes appear to blink, flinch, or change their gaze. They are mute and show no signs of conscious awareness; hence, the common textbook description of "awake but not aware." They are incontinent of urine and feces, cannot feed themselves, and despite media legends to the contrary, they never wake up and go home. To use a modern metaphor, these terrible victims are medical zombies who may give the illusion of self-awareness and emotionality but seem entirely bereft of these precious human traits.

But this tidy neurological category has become murkier in recent years, stirring up troubling doubts among families and the medical community that diagnoses these tragic victims.

Occasionally, a person classified as in a persistent vegetative state may show some outward signs of conscious awareness. One day, after months or years of keeping a silent vigil, they may utter a meaningful phrase, purposefully reach for an object, or smile deliberately at a loved one. Their functional brain MRI scans start to show glowing ambers of activity where there was once only darkness. This condition is now referred to as a minimally conscious state (MCS). Rarely is there any further improvement, but the haunting question is raised: When can we be sure that conscious awareness has been fully extinguished, is still present, or may someday return? How can we ever know if there is still a person "inside there" like Joe's mother asked?

The room featured typical nursing home décor. Tan or light-yellow painted walls, hospital-style bed, and a large cork board covered with photos of family—children at various stages of life; a brown-haired wife; a tall, muscular husband; winter sleds; and summer swimming pools. Joe was sitting up in a large maroon chair. Staring blankly ahead, with the feeding tube hidden under an oversized Penn State sweatshirt, one might mistake him for a contemplative person enjoying a few minutes of solitude. I imagined him pulling the sled upward on that snowy day in the photo, his children squealing, "Faster, Daddy, real fast!" or splashing water in the pool with his bikini-clad wife one July afternoon years ago.

But Joe is mute, motionless, *awake but not aware*, I later wrote in my consult note. He does not follow with his eyes, does not flinch or withdraw a limb with a pin stick ("noxious stimuli" is the medical euphemism). He does not answer questions or follow a simple command. The only outward sign that something very grave has happened to him is the craniotomy scar along the right side of his head, visible through his thinning but combed hair. His brain scans and EEG results do not underscore his clinical presentation. Some residual scar tissue in the right hemisphere visible on MRI, and the EEG tracing shows some mild slowing in brain wave rhythms—the same it might show if you became drowsy during a less-than-inspiring lecture or movie.

"Will he wake up, Doctor? Will he be a prisoner forever?" the mother asked. I noticed that Joe had her brown-green eyes and thick nose.

"Joe has already woken up," I stated bluntly. "But this is probably the best he'll ever be, and there is no evidence that I can see that he has any self-awareness or awareness of his surroundings. Spend time with him, talk to him. We can never really know for sure. Maybe he understands more than we realize."

I regretted the last line. Her eyes flared and her pupils dilated. She felt justification for the countless hours, changing his diapers, adjusting the feeding tube, bathing him, giving him updates about his children. *Maybe, maybe he hears and listens and understands. Maybe.*

Did I encourage her delusion? Give her false hope? Was I professionally negligent? Who's to say? Consciousness may be the ultimate scientific mystery. A first-person impenetrable phenomenon. I explained to her about irreversible brain injury and the statistically negligible possibility of him showing *any* improvement after all this time. But all she heard was the "maybe."

Before I left the premises, I walked by Joe's room again. Two teenage children were standing over him, one showing him some soccer game footage on her iPhone. Their conversation was animated. Joe stared blankly ahead, quiet…listening?

Maybe…

Anna O. Redux

A prevailing modern notion, buttressed partially by science, is that the universe and everything that happens in it—including all human activity—is merely the consequence of chance and necessity, and this notion has become more widely accepted in our digital age. The philosophical opposite—that everything is deterministic and all events are inevitably governed by the laws of nature (or an omniscient god)—seems equally extreme. Both views are fatalistic, leaving little room for that most precious gift of human nature: free will. Modern brain science seems to lend credence to this pessimistic state of affairs by offering up supposed evidence that our brains are constantly running unconscious programs that govern everything from our moods to our beliefs and our very emotions, even love. Yes, the human brain can be partially likened to an incredibly complex computer, but that by no means indicates that human free will is an illusion and that our deterministic fates are sealed like automatons. As in all human affairs, nothing is ever exactly what it seems. And the human mind is no exception.

Anna T. had recently lost her father to liver cancer, and as a result her mother moved in with her. This was partially good news because Anna had recently separated from her husband over financial issues (multiple failed business ventures, she would later explain to me) and needed help with her two young sons, taking care of the house, and all the daily chores necessary to running a home. By all accounts, she was a bright and responsible young mom seemingly in good health, but she recently had been prone to episodes of crying. She felt overwhelmed by her failing marriage, the death of a parent, and the relentless duties, financial and otherwise, of modern parenting. One November morning, she awoke and realized that she could not negotiate her way out of bed. She first struggled with adjusting her arms and torso until she realized that she could not feel or move the dead weight below her hips. Her legs were paralyzed.

The children, still asleep, did not hear her scream. She called out to her mother who ran into the bedroom. At first, they both thought that maybe her legs were simply numb from a deep sleep. Her mom rubbed Anna's feet and legs and tried to cajole them back to life, but it didn't work. Anna remained eerily calm. She slowly explained to her mom that she needed to call 911. "You'll have to stay here with the kids. When they wake up, fix them breakfast and just tell them I had to go to the hospital for a checkup and I'll be back later."

Acute paraplegia in a young person is always a portentous diagnosis. Malignant spinal cord and brain tumors, strokes, physical trauma, and even viral infections are all possible suspects. When something so dramatic happens so quickly to the body, the outcome is often not good. Time is crucial in these scenarios because the longer the cause goes undetected, the more likely the damage will be permanent. The fear of medical malpractice always looms large in such high-risk cases as well. Before I arrived at the ER, the staff had already called neurosurgery and arranged for stat brain and spine MRIs. They would prove to be entirely normal as would the subsequent spinal tap. The young Ivy League-trained neurosurgeon already signed off on the case. "Nothing surgical here, no tumor, no herniated disc, no bleed," he dismissively announced and then added, "Sounds like a real 'fascinoma' just for you, Dr. A."

Fascinoma is the pejorative medical colloquialism for a case that seems unusual but will often turn out to be something ordinary, or at least something not at all strange. At this point, the hospital staff was viewing Anna with some suspicion. Was she really that sick? After all, all these sophisticated diagnostic tests were normal. I walked into her exam room and pulled the curtains closed.

"Hi, Anna. I'm the neurologist on call this evening. The ER staff asked me to take a look at you. I understand the trouble started this morning when you woke up, right?"

"I was perfectly fine yesterday. Like I told the other doctors, I haven't been sick, no fevers, no recent back injuries, nothing at all."

"What seems to be troubling you the most?"

"I can't move my legs at all, I can't even feel them. I mean, there's no pain or anything. I just woke up like this. Will it get better soon?" Her demeanor remained detached as if she didn't have a care in the world.

"The good news is that all the diagnostic tests are entirely normal. That means there's no evidence of stroke, tumor, infection, or other life-threatening diseases. This doesn't mean that there isn't a serious neurological problem. It just means that we haven't uncovered it yet." That was the fairest response I could provide to her at this time.

"Do you have any family history of similar problems with your parents or siblings—things like seizure disorders or unusual unexplained behavior?"

"No, Doctor, we're all pretty healthy except for my father dying from liver cancer."

"And your two sons?"

"They're very healthy, do good in school too. My mom helps with them; she lives with us. Doctor, I'm kind of hungry now, can I get something to eat?"

For the next several days, she remained bed stricken in the neurology ward. The physical therapists came by daily and worked with her. They passively moved her legs through exercises to avoid further deconditioning, but her legs remained dead weight. She relieved herself using a bed pan and spent much time watching daytime TV cooking shows.

One morning I stopped by while I was making hospital rounds. Anna was crying in her bed. The psychiatrist had just visited her, at my request. He diagnosed her with reactive depression and placed her on a standard antidepressant medication as is common in patients hospitalized with major neurological problems.

"Today, I'd like to see if we can get some movement in those legs of yours. Your complete spinal fluid results have returned, and they're perfectly normal as were the rest of your MRI scans that we repeated, just to make sure we're not missing anything. This is good news, you know."

Anna gave a faint smile. "Sometimes everything is just too much for me; there's too much happening. The kids, the bills, my father dying. I'm pretty much on my own now; my mom does all she can, but not having a husband around has taken its toll on all of us. I started having panic attacks over the past couple of months, and now this." She pointed to her legs.

"I can imagine," I said sympathetically. "Let's see if you can muster enough willpower to move one of those legs, or maybe just a foot."

Her eyes squinted and her face contorted like she was trying to lift a ponderously heavy weight.

"No, don't overdo it. Just relax and concentrate on your feet. How about just the toes for now?"

And with that, she tentatively, and then briskly, wiggled all her toes on both feet.

I smiled. "Hard part is over."

As I walked down the hallway, I smiled again, but this time

to myself. How much of our precious free will, that sacred legacy of billions of neurons, is real? At any given moment our brains are busy working countless tasks without any self-awareness on our part—controlling heart and breathing rates, subtle adjustments in pituitary and kidney function, changes in eye movement, postural body changes, and maybe even our very thoughts before we know them or have words before we speak them. How much of human behavior is on autopilot?

Anna struggled with physical therapy for three months but eventually made a full recovery and was able to walk normally. When she came to my office for a follow-up visit, she was optimistic but cautious. Her life resumed where it had paused before the illness, and she was seeing a psychologist for counseling. She asked me earnestly, "Doctor, what really happened to me?"

About a century ago, the legendary psychiatrist (and neurologist) Sigmund Freud wrote about another Anna, known as Anna O. She was a bright, intellectual young lady who enjoyed all the amenities of her privileged Victorian life. At the age of twenty she began experiencing episodes of sudden paralysis of her right arm and leg. Convinced that this was not the result of stroke, seizure, or other neurological disease, she was subjected to hypnosis (fashionable at the time) and elicited painful repressed memories of cradling her dying father with her right arm. Once she gained insight into this matter, she was presumably able to resume a normal life again. Such conditions are referred to as conversion disorders. The term is a legacy of the Freudian view that all abnormal human behavior can be explained in terms of unconscious motives and conflicts. Conversion disorders typically present with sudden and dramatic neurological symptoms such as acute blindness or sudden paralysis. The ancient Greeks used the term "hysteria" when describing similar conditions. They invoked the notion of a "wandering uterus" as an explanation to why more women than men seemed to suffer from such conditions. In the Middle Ages, such odd behavior, as well as epilepsy, was chalked up to demonic possession. It was not until the renowned nineteenth-century French neurologist Jean-Martin Charcot turned a scientific eye toward this enigma and speculated that these patients suffered from a degenerative neurological disease that was triggered by a traumatic emotional event. This paved the way for the Freudian interpretation of conversion disorder as a symbolic expression of an unconscious psychological conflict, which he elucidated after studying Anna O.

In this early view, then, a conversion disorder really is just a metaphor the mind creates, a representation of an unconscious fear or experience. A woman who suspects her husband's infidelity may suddenly become "blind," or a mother who could not rescue her drowning child becomes "paraplegic." The radioactive glow on modern PET scans now show physical changes in the limbic lobes of the brains of such people.

And what of our Anna? A tidy little explanation eluded me. She was a young woman under some stress but clearly did not suffer any profound psychiatric malady. About two years later, she came back to see me in my office. She was doing well and her children were thriving. She had been experiencing some leg cramping, which appeared to be a minor muscle spasm. You see, in response to her "experience" as she called it, she had taken up marathon running and was becoming regionally known for her exceptional performance in several amateur meets. She told me, "When I got sick, I felt like I had no control over myself; I felt like my mind had hijacked my body. I never want to feel that way again."

None of us ever want to. I smiled, this time outwardly. That's what the struggle to be human is all about.

The Premature Burial

I HAD TO look up the proper term in my psychiatric glossary, which contains a seemingly endless list of phobias and the appropriate jargon used to describe them. The fear of being buried alive is called "taphephobia," which literally translates as "fear of graves." That primal fear has long been the staple of horror stories and movies ever since Edgar Allan Poe's original tales, which I had not read since high school. My patient seemed to have an encyclopedic knowledge on the subject of being buried alive. He knew of all the historical references. Vestal virgins were buried alive in ancient Rome for presumably violating their celibacy. The Japanese buried Chinese enemies alive during World War II. Even George Washington, he eagerly told me as if taking pride in the renowned company he shared his condition with, was anxious about a premature grave and asked that he be kept in his bed for a couple of days before burial to be certain he was really dead. My patient's knowledge of the subject was impressive. He explained that throughout history, particularly medieval and Victorian, there was somewhat of a cultural obsession regarding premature burials. He was a community college history professor, never married, and devoted to his profession. Physically healthy and in his early forties, he, however, had concerns.

He was always a "nervous type" as he described himself. He said that his mother often referred to him as "the worried tadpole" when he was growing up. He spent much of his childhood reading history, as his love for the subject began in grade school. Always thin, frail, pale, and short in stature (perhaps calling to mind a tadpole?), he avoided most typical teenage activities like sports and girls. A perpetual insomniac, he was treated for mild depression and anxiety on and off for most of his adult life.

He had come to see me after suffering a "spell" of sorts. Just before he was to start one of his routine history lectures at the college, he inexplicably began feeling very anxious. Sitting in a faculty lounge with some colleagues, he could feel his palms becoming sweaty and his heart pounding, and he struggled to catch his breath. Mere indigestion? No. Maybe a heart attack? Imminent stroke? All these fears started circling as his mind raced uncontrollably, his vision blurred, and his hands started to tingle. He excused himself to rush to the bathroom but quickly collapsed over his chair. He regained full consciousness with a splash of water on his face as he was helped back into his chair, mortified by the experience. On the insistence of his fellow professors, 911 was called and he was whisked off to the local hospital ER. There he promptly underwent the routine investigation for such episodes: electrocardiogram, brain CAT scan, blood tests, and urine toxicology (to make certain the good professor wasn't abusing drugs like cocaine or amphetamines, he wasn't). The emergency room doctors suggested that he may have suffered a panic attack. He was given an appointment to follow up with a neurologist (me) to make certain of the diagnosis.

In my office the professor explained to me how he may have suffered similar episodes over the course of his adult life and that they had been relatively uncommon. He also admitted being treated for mild depression in the past. I reviewed his various test results and concluded that he had indeed suffered a classic panic attack. Typically, in these kinds of cases, once I conclude that there is no neurological problem, I promptly refer the patient to a psychiatrist to consider drug treatment for depression and anxiety, two conditions that commonly coexist in people who suffer panic disorders. In this case, however, I was intrigued by his newfound historical interest in premature burials.

In fact, his panic attack occurred moments before he was to give a lecture discussing the frenzied preoccupation of untimely burials during the eighteenth and nineteenth centuries, particularly in Victorian England.

He explained to me that a variety of devices had been invented and patented to allow a living person to signal to the outside world should he or she awaken and find themselves accidentally entombed—devices that would allow the unfortunate victim to ring a bell, for instance, which would connect to a pulley leading to the surface. Pipelines would allow the unobstructed flow of air to the grave as well to prevent slow asphyxiation from lack of air, a particularly gruesome demise but perhaps not as bad as slowly dehydrating from lack of water. Some of these "safety coffins" as they were called even had provisions of food and water in small compartments for the "undead" to enjoy while awaiting rescue! For those wealthy enough to afford above-ground accommodations, various means were created to allow for detection of any signs of life in the entombed, including windows, pulley devices, and sound amplifiers to detect breath sounds. More recent devices in this century included electronic electrocardiograms to detect heartbeats. It may all seem very macabre, but the possibility of being buried while still alive, although appearing lifeless, was not so remote at least a century or two ago. There are several neurological conditions that could mimic death, to an untrained eye, in an otherwise healthy person. Like most phobias, there was some basis in reality for his fears, or at least there could have been a century ago.

A person who is about to suffer a sudden seizure may appear perfectly normal, perhaps in the midst of a conversation, before he or she suddenly collapses to the ground, convulsing uncontrollably with arms and legs twitching and flailing while totally unconscious. After a few minutes the convulsing may stop and labored breathing may follow, with the victim still unarousable. The person would appear lifeless for minutes to hours depending on the severity of the seizure in this postictal state. Imagine a young woman, who at the sudden site of blood—perhaps a bloody limb laceration on one of her children—suddenly collapses to the ground and lies unconscious. This simple faint (or "vasovagal syncope" to use the technical term) is quite common. Many of us have experienced such syncope (or at least a near-faint) often triggered by sudden pain, fear, or emotional stress. Usually, the person will awaken fully coherent if not a little embarrassed within a minute or less, but until then he or she may appear still and lifeless.

Cataplexy and its neurological cousin narcolepsy also may mimic death very dramatically. In cataplexy, a sudden emotion such as fear, laughter, or excitement can trigger sudden loss of muscle tone, collapse, and unconsciousness for several minutes. One young patient learned of her cataplexy for the first time when she collapsed after entering her college dormitory room only to be surprised by a birthday party. In narcolepsy, people often fall asleep instantly, sometimes in midsentence during a conversation.

Now the professor suffered none of these ailments as far as I could tell, but he knew about them. They worried him. Simple reassurances didn't help. I explained to him that today, in the twenty-first century, all of these conditions and others were widely recognized. I explained that I was aware of no recorded misdiagnosis where a living person was thought to be dead and then buried alive. Again I explained that like all dreaded phobias, this one had some rational basis in reality but was bizarrely exaggerated in this instance.

Weeks later he began having nightmares. They were not the

ordinary kind that we all have experienced, where we awaken and realize it was only a frightening dream. He would thrash about the bed, knocking over a night table lamp and pulling out blanket and sheets saturated with his perspiration, and awaken horrified. In his dreams he was buried alive, trying to claw his way out of his wood coffin, granite tomb, or subterranean crypt, depending on which of the multiple variations of the nightmare he was having. (Such a condition where one physically acts out during a nightmare is known as REM sleep disorder and is common.) He became an insomniac for fear of sleeping and dreaming. He stopped lecturing about the history of premature burials because even talking about the topic made him nervous. Finally, with my advice again, he relented and saw a psychiatrist. He was placed on some antianxiety medication, as well as a sedative drug to take at bedtime. His symptoms improved slightly; at least he could sleep three or four hours per night. But he was still tormented. Here was this relatively young, successful academic who was gradually becoming a psychological invalid because of a singular phobia that was consuming him. He wasn't insane or deranged, and in most other spheres of his life, he could function normally. Unlike other phobias that I have encountered in patients—fear of heights, fear of public speaking, fear of closed or confined spaces—this fear was particularly insidious. He started losing weight and was not eating well. He began seeing a therapist

I imagined a simple thought experiment: If I hooked him up to a PET brain scan and started reading a passage from one of his lectures about premature burials (or showed him depictions of such), his amygdalae (right and left) would light up like a Christmas tree. These are the primordial brain structures that mediate fear and its relevant emotional content.

Several months went by and I presumed that I would never see him again, as his problems were really not neurological in the sense that I could not provide him with any direct medical treatment. But one morning he returned to my office. He looked better and said he was sleeping easier and had regained his appetite. He was still taking a mild antianxiety medication but was no longer seeing his psychotherapist. I was rather surprised; phobias don't just resolve spontaneously.

"I've been doing much better, Dr. Adamo," he said in a sanguine tone.

"What about the nightmares, your preoccupation with…" I was careful not to use the words "burial," "premature," or "death."

"You know, you have to confront your fears, stare the abyss directly in its face," he answered. "I thought the problem through, and I came to a solution which really has gone a long way in alleviating my fear, or preoccupation."

I was intrigued and nodded as he went on to explain.

"You know how people with heart conditions or diabetes or dangerous allergies wear those medical alert bracelets, so in case of an emergency doctors and nurses will know a person's medical background if you can't tell them, like if you're unconscious or in some kind of coma?"

I nodded yes.

"Well, I got one of those bracelets, and I always wear it around my right wrist. I also have a medical info card that I keep in my wallet."

"What kind of information do you have on it? You don't have any of those medical problems."

He grinned and showed me his bracelet. The inscription read:

> In case of my demise all funeral services must be delayed for a full 120 hours after death is medically determined. Thank you and godspeed!

"I figure that's enough time. If I haven't woken up by then, I probably won't ever."

The Remains

The stream of consciousness that constitutes the movie of each life is seamless. There are no jump-edits or abrupt cuts as long as the brain engine can greedily feed on its energy. The brain consumes glucose and oxygen relentlessly; a few minutes without one or both and the great miracle of mind awareness collapses into darkness. Coma, persistent vegetative state, minimally conscious state, and brain death are the vernacular of my trade, each specifying something catastrophic has happened. Some of these diagnoses are escapable and the movie can resume; others are forever.

We often hear and speak platitudes about how precious life is and how we should count each day as a gift. Many of us cannot imagine their true import. An occupational hazard of the physician is the recognition that seemingly good health and youthful vigor can be illusory. A fateful miscoding of a DNA sequence in your cells may stir growth of a malignant brain tumor, a microscopic piece of sludge in a coronary artery may lethally quiver your heart, or a segment of an aneurysmal brain artery may stretch out like a child's bursting bubblegum and explode.

Sometimes all the physician can offer is to act as navigator for the bereaved as they travel the uncharted territory of shock and grief. All ancient and modern cultures—Neolithic, Mesopotamian, Egyptian, Greek, Christian, Muslim—had or have rites and rituals to guide the living and the dead. Modern medicine often replaces religious practice with its own sterile protocols, especially if the end of life occurs in the hospital, an inevitable fate for many of us.

Jack and Emma were happy enough. A successful Wall Street career kept Jack's wife and two healthy preteen children well provided for: a big colonial in a good school district, a loving family life, and a stable marriage. Their lives were enviable, and most would agree that it doesn't get any better than this. His recent headaches were attributed to the stress of a high-powered financial career, or maybe it was just some jet lag having returned from a family trip to the Caribbean. One night a loud thud awoke his wife; Jack lay on the bathroom floor seizing with his arms flexed. By the time the medics arrived, he was motionless.

"Call Neurology, now! Unresponsive to all stimuli and unarousable. Let's get a brain CT, but first I have to intubate him; he's barely breathing." The ER staff was in a whirlwind of activity. A young man gravely sick is not the kind of case you want to falter on. You don't want tragedy on your shoulders, or a malpractice case for that matter. And so my home phone rang at 2:00 a.m.

"Forty-two-year-old man, intubated on life support, collapsed at home with witnessed seizure, brain CT/CTA shows subarachnoid hemorrhage with clotted PCOM aneurysm. I called neurosurgery, but I don't think there's much they can do for him." I listened to the disembodied voice as I was jarred out of sleep.

By the time I arrived, patient Jack Lormenti, read the ID bracelet, was already in the ICU. After I examined him, I found his wife. She was seated in a small room with a couch, dimly lit with a traditional table lamp, which seemed very out of place in the ICU. The room was labeled "Consultation and Meditation Area." This is the place were typically most people hear bad news.

I motioned to the wife to sit on the couch, and I sat down first. I imagined her children waiting at home, wide awake now in the middle of a school night. Maybe a grandparent was summoned to watch them.

"Your husband has a massive brain hemorrhage from a ruptured cerebral aneurysm. The aneurysm has been there, maybe for most of his life. Unfortunately, we often do not know what we carry inside ourselves. Oftentimes these aneurysms rupture suddenly and without warning. Do you know if he had been complaining of any symptoms, such as headaches? Is there anyone in his family—siblings, parents—with a history of brain aneurysms?"

She shook her head no. "He sometimes would get headaches, but they were no big deal…He would take Tylenol and he'd be fine."

I continued, "You see, right now he is in a deep coma, even his breathing and blood pressure have to be maintained with life support. The neurosurgeon doesn't think he would survive a craniotomy, you know, to drain the blood and repair the ruptured blood vessel."

"What should I tell the children?" she whispered.

"Let's wait a day or so and see what happens, but I can't honestly hold out any real optimism for you based on the way things look right now."

I remember thinking there's a medical term for this: "therapeutic nihilism." I could offer no real hope of treatment or even improvement. Even aggressive brain surgeons have to turn their backs on some cases. All you can do is help the living navigate a pathway, at best, where there is really none to begin with.

I imagined the wife arriving back at home that night. It's late and the kids are in bed, but they're wide awake. They're worried. "How's Dad? When is he coming home?" they ask nervously. They might not be old enough to grasp the ephemeral nature of things. Parents and family and home are supposed to be immutable. Things just don't collapse. Why would something like this happen? There's no reason for it; it isn't fair. Maybe, they wonder, this is a punishment for some imagined wrong they committed.

"Dad's very sick. He's in a coma, and the doctors don't

know if he'll wake up or not."

"Will he have to stay in the hospital for always then, Mom?"

"No, sweetie, he'll go to heaven."

"Then will the doctors in heaven make him better?"

"No, sweetie, it doesn't work that way."

"Won't Dad miss us in heaven? Won't he get lonely?"

"In heaven everyone is happy, dear."

"Jamie Carter in my class says his parents don't believe in heaven. They told him that when you die, there's just nothing like you were never even born, and it's peaceful."

I smiled to myself—a child's innocent logic trying to unravel the conundrum of eternal oblivion vs. eternal life.

A day passed and I sat again with the wife, this time bedside next to her husband and the mechanical respirator that was heaving and humming. The machine watched over him, forcing the chest to rise and infusing some deceptive lifelike color into his swollen face.

"He looks better, Doctor; I think he can hear my voice, maybe."

"I know things may appear that way, but from a neurological point of view, that's not happening." I didn't mention the term brain death, yet. I responded as neutrally as possible.

"I'm sorry, but I believe there's been some further deterioration in his condition. Remember what we talked about the other day. Your husband suffered a ruptured brain aneurysm, and the damage was catastrophic. Now, with the passage of some time, we can see that the brain injury is permanent, irreversible. He no longer possesses even the most basic brain-stem abilities—breathing on his own, heart rate control, or blood pressure regulation. Even the most basic brain stem functions are lost. We know that he can never recover from this state; there will never be any conscious awareness. He is no longer alive in any sense. He meets all the neurological criteria for what we call brain death. He is, in reality, dead, only for the machines does his heart keep pumping blood and his lungs continue filling with air."

She averted her eyes from me, as if to deny the ugly reality that I brought to her. "But his face has some color in it, his blood tests are all normal. How can he be dead?" she sobbed quietly.

The harvesters soon came. There was little time. A young healthy man struck down before his prime. His organs were healthy—a strong heart, clean nonsmoker lungs, good kidneys, unscarred corneas. This team of doctors and nurses, all organ-transplant experts, had the unenviable task of convincing a grieving spouse or parent to give up the vital organs of their loved one. There is certain altruism in this endeavor as young lives can be saved with the death of a young life. Often, however, the harvesters are greeted with suspicion and resentment by the bereaved. There is, after all, a touch of the macabre in all of it. "Why should someone benefit from the death of my husband?"

"The hospital will just let him die so they can get his organs; it's all big business!" "What about his soul? What will become of that if you take out his heart and give it to someone else?" Often families will overcome their suspicions or superstitions and see the generous nobility in organ donation. Lives can be saved, often a child's life. Some see it as providing meaning to an otherwise senseless death or even achieving a kind of immortality.

The brain-dead man's wife agreed to organ donation—his lungs and kidneys; she hesitated on the heart. The harvesters wanted it all; each vital morsel is a life saved.

The next morning, the children made an appearance in their father's ICU room. They were spared discussions of brain death and organ transplants, The mother had simply explained that this might be the last time they would see their father. The daughter wrapped a brightly colored, homemade string bracelet around her dad's right wrist. The son tried to hold back his sobbing.

When the mother and children left the room, I watched them walk down the white ICU corridor. The staff swept into the room and the organ procurement ritual began. The breathing machine heaved; his chest rose as if alive. The surgeons began scrubbing their hands. The harvesters were eagerly waiting.

A dying child would be saved by his heart, another by his liver. His corneas would give sight to a young man. And one of his lungs would breathe life into a dying teenager.

But no one removed the daughter's string bracelet. The family insisted on that.

Man Plans...

He was a young lawyer, as was his wife: Rob and Jen, both in their late twenties. She was about six weeks pregnant with their first child when I first met them. Their plan was to have at least three. They purchased a nice-sized colonial on an acre, big enough to accommodate their future family. Their careers were just starting to gain steam, and they were building a secure financial future. There would be plenty of money for family vacations to Disney World, college funds, and retirement.

There's an old Yiddish adage: *Mann traoch, Gott lauch* (Man plans, God laughs). The saying is supposed to imply not the cruel nature of a diabolical god but the inherent unpredictability of our fragile lives and plans.

Six months after the initial diagnosis

"At Sloan they're saying one of the three bigger lesions might be about half a millimeter smaller in diameter. They might even extend the radiation therapy to a few extra sessions, but I told them no. I've had two brain surgeries, three trials of the chemo and the radiation. I know they've done all they can, and now that's it," Rob explains to me in a matter-of-fact tone. "I just want to be home with Jen the next few months."

About six months earlier, Rob presented to my office for what seemed to be a minor issue. He had been noticing "cramps" in his left calf, especially when playing basketball with his buddies or running on the treadmill. His family doctor promptly sent him for a knee X-ray and prescribed some muscle relaxants, having diagnosed him with a muscle sprain. But Rob suspected something more, as he explained, "Sometimes my leg would just shake uncontrollably for about a minute, jerking back and forth." He was describing to me focal motor seizures, brief involuntary jerks of a limb. The brain MRI showed a large angry-looking mass, the size of a baseball with another two smaller masses, the total size of a golf ball. It looked like he had more tumor than brain in his skull. And yet, he sat comfortably in my office, speaking eloquently about a seemingly minor symptom that really only interfered with his basketball game. Tall and athletic-looking, he was expecting to be told that he merely was suffering a muscle sprain. But in my office on this day, this bright autumn day in September, he's looking somewhat emaciated and wearing a baseball cap that conceals his shaven scalp and the large, right-sided surgical wound with the bright metallic staples still in place.

"They told me I can expect about three to six more months at best, which means I'll probably still be around when Jen gives birth. That's all I want now, to see this through, the birth of our child, and whatever comes after that, well…" His voice quivers and he stops talking.

They call this the acceptance stage of dying or grieving or both. It seems more like resignation, I think. It's not resignation born of apathy but rather a heroic submission to the inevitable.

Four months after the initial diagnosis

"I don't see the point in all of this. It's malignant, the most malignant brain tumor you can get—glioblastoma, that's what they call it. I'm getting the radiation therapy, chemo too, had one brain surgery, and their scheduling a second one soon. Debulking, that's what they call it? What's the point? All you docs have already told me that the survival rate is about fifteen months for this damn thing."

Rob is somber but still looks healthy. His hair is growing back, slowly covering his surgical wound over his head. He's lost only a little weight and the steroids give him a ruddy complexion, which could be mistaken for a healthy glow. He continues, this time sarcastically, "What's the point? I mean why don't I just take a trip with Jen? Maybe go to Disney; after all, the three of us may never make it there again." His eyes swell up.

I feel as if there's a gusher behind them waiting to flood the room with his misery. He's angry, miserable, and depressed all at once. But he's also hopeful, though he doesn't want to let me, or himself, on to it.

The stages of dying are supposed to be neat and tidy, but of course the medical school model that we were taught is only a sketchy roadmap for the dark landscape of grief. First there's supposed to be denial. The patient-victim cannot accept or even assimilate the dreaded diagnosis. There must be some kind of mistake, some misunderstanding. This will all turn out to be false. The doctors will realize this soon enough. Taken to its pathological extreme, this fixed delusion can become psychosis, but typically this stage gives way to anger.

With anger, the individual can masquerade with a mock strength, at least temporarily. The textbooks say Rob should now be in the depression stage. But real life is a lot messier.

"Recently I had to purchase a dehumidifier. I've always had allergies, and we keep one running in the basement," he explained to me one day during an office visit. "In the store, the cashier asked me if I wanted to buy the extended warranty—two-, three-, or four-year duration. I didn't know what to say… we take so much for granted."

Three weeks after the initial diagnosis

"Listen, Rob, you've already had three medical opinions from three different neurosurgeons, all of whom specialize in brain tumor oncology. All the opinions are unanimous. The tumor must be removed. There's no hope without the surgery." I explain this as patiently as I can to him, but I know that with such an aggressive cancer, a few weeks may cut down on his already limited survival rate.

"But, Doc, I'm going to start some changes. I'll eat better, go vegetarian. And I'm starting a vitamin regimen. We know a nutritionist. I've been exercising too. I've read that all of this will build up my immune system. I know you think some of this might be crazy, but let's give it a few weeks and see." Rob is a lawyer and perhaps his default mode is to take the Socratic method and negotiate his case. Perhaps try to convince me that somehow I, and three leading specialists, have all made a logical misstep. I'll try to reason with him, but I know what this is. It's called the bargaining stage. I've seen two approaches to this over the years.

The first is the sacred view. One will negotiate with God. The person will view the terminal diagnosis as some kind of cosmic punishment. It is a warning that he or she must reform their ways by living a more humane lifestyle, more religious, more compassionate. One must atone for whatever perceived transgressions one has committed. This will make things right and perhaps offer a way out of the incurable diagnosis. The second approach is more secular and not based on any religious presuppositions. This was Rob's approach and not surprising given his more agnostic worldview. He was desperately trying to take refuge in the prominent pseudoscientific fallacy of our age: diet, exercise, and vitamins, in all the right amounts, can stave off any disease and maybe even death. It puts the patient seemingly back in control, when in reality there may be none.

"Rob, listen to me," I say, staring directly at him across my desk. "You can't fix this problem with diet and vitamins and running a marathon. This is not a lifestyle problem. You already lead a healthy lifestyle. You don't smoke, drink, or engage in any reckless behavior. This is an unlucky hand in the deck of cards. You know that."

"I know, Doc, I know," he whispers back.

Two weeks after the initial diagnosis

The stages of dying—denial, anger, bargaining, depression, and finally acceptance—represent a general framework that can apply to any adversity one is confronted with in life. In reality, the stages are really a roadmap that varies, has twists and turns, and can go back and forth without being linear. About two weeks after Rob learned that there was a malignant cancer growing inside his head, he started to show that predictable anger, masking his fear and sadness. With his young wife at his side, he protested: "How can this be? Damn this. I never smoked cigarettes or did drugs. My parents are healthy. I'm young. I have so much that I need to do! We're gonna have a family; my career is doing really well. How is this even possible?"

His wife, stoic and rational, or at least trying to be, would try to redirect his energy. "Rob, please let's just focus on what we need to do next to keep you moving forward."

His eyes well up with tears, the only time I've ever seen him cry during the entire ordeal.

The week of the initial diagnosis

"Hi, Rob, I was hoping to discuss this in person rather than a phone call, but I have the brain MRI results. We can discuss this, but you should also come in soon," I say, trying not to betray any real emotion. This brief conversation would soon shatter his life.

"Doc, the radiologist gave me copies of the films. I know I'm not trained in reading these things, but I can see big white blotches in the right half of the MRI and smaller white blotches in the left." He tries to sound objective and gives a nervous chuckle.

"Rob, those 'blotches' represent the tumor. It looks quite malignant. This is what we talked about. You'll need to see neurosurgery. The lesions will have to be biopsied."

"Doc, aren't you getting ahead of yourself? I mean I really don't feel that bad. This could be anything, right? You know I had a couple of concussions back when I played ball in college. Maybe that's what we're seeing now?" His voice wavers.

The next day he's in my office for an appointment. His wife is with him this time. It is the first time I meet her. She's young and slender and volunteers that she is a few weeks pregnant with their first child. Rob's mood is somewhat elated. He hasn't slept in a couple of days. I try to imagine what it must be like to be in his shoes. Young, full of promise and life, only to be told that he will be robbed of everything he has planned and hoped for in his life. There is a tumor—not in a convenient location like the liver, lung, or kidney, all places where such an abomination could perhaps be excised and dealt with efficiently. No, this tumor is in the brain, the very center of the universe that houses the mind, memory, and self. With each surgical resection and each irradiation, pieces of the mind, memory, and self will be destroyed. Today, we won't discuss this. But we will soon enough. Today, we'll discuss clinical technicalities such as neurosurgery, biopsies, and treatment options. I'll avoid the real questions like survival rates and quality of life and "How long do I have?" I'll be diplomatic and clever: "Well, we'll need to see what the pathology is after the biopsy. Some tumors are very treatable." This is true enough, but this young man has a head full of cancer. "Let's wait and see," I'll tell him. I'm being compassionate, I think, but he's still not ready to hear the truth.

He will live to see the birth of his daughter but not her first birthday.

Tomorrowland

The eternal now is forever fleeting, and the future does not yet exist. It is the past that makes us who we are. Our unique memories and past experiences are stored and encoded in our brain, a fragile web made up of billions of neurons with trillions of connections, once referred to as an "enchanted loom." Someday, maybe, we will be able to upload our memories, thoughts, and experiences from our brains onto something more permanent like a computer disc or artificial intelligence machine, perhaps attaining some kind of immortality. Until then, the enchanted loom is fragile and impermanent.

It was a sunny spring day and the old man decided to take a little trip. He grabbed a sweater, a small orange, and a blue-colored map and headed for the Flushing Meadows Corona Park in Queens, New York City. Confused about the park's exact location, he knew enough to take the Long Island Rail Road west to Jamaica station, and from there, with the kindness of strangers, he got subway directions. He stopped along the way and purchased a Hershey's chocolate bar at the grocery store, intending to save it for the trip back home. When he finally arrived at the park, he was surprised to see it mostly empty. He noticed a man walking a dog and a jogger or two, but he expected a much larger crowd for a Wednesday morning. He made his way to the giant Unisphere and was the solitary figure under the enormous and elegant steel globe. He recognized the New York State Pavilion, looking strangely dilapidated, and trekked briskly over to it, but once again he found himself alone under the bright sunlight.

He eventually sat down on a park bench and ate the Hershey's bar. The looming towers grew shadowy, and the sun eventually started to fade. By now he was getting a little anxious. He knew darkness would soon follow the twilight. He waved to a young runner and showed her his map, crumbled but legible: Welcome to the World's Fair 1964–65 at Flushing Meadows.

"I'm trying to find the Progressland. I think it's at the General Electric Pavilion. Where the hell is everybody? The damn place is so big!" he exclaimed to the lady, too young to even imagine what ancient history the old man was referencing.

The GE Pavilion would be just due east of his location on the park bench, a few hundred feet past Polynesia, IBM, Dupont, and the Tower of Lights. But that was over fifty years ago.

The jogger called 911. The police and an ambulance arrived shortly.

"It started about a year ago," the daughter explained. "You know we just attributed it to old age. He's almost ninety and in good shape otherwise. A little confusion around the house, we don't let him drive anymore, and my mom handles the bills now. Then one day he disappears and we get a call from Queen's General, and they tell us he's in the ER, picked up roaming around Corona Park. They did some blood tests and a CAT scan of the brain, but everything was normal."

It's a familiar story, especially these days with the aging demographics around our country. I reviewed the medical records and went through my routine mental status exam, adding up and subtracting points for orientation, registration, recall, language, judgments, general cognition, etc. It was mostly a moot academic exercise, for the family's benefit, to provide the imprimatur of science on what they already knew. He knew the month April, but not the date or the year, and confidently said the president was Lyndon B. Johnson. This was all consistent with Alzheimer's disease.

I asked my patient, Joe Sardone, what he was doing that day all the way in Queens, far from his home in central Long Island.

"Doc, all I wanted is to take another look at the World's Fair. It used to be beautiful. We took the whole family there—sons, daughters, the wife. It was the future, boy, and I never forgot the Progressland. But it's gone…I knew it would be." He whispered the last phrase with a kind of self-aware irony like he ultimately knew he would never find what he was looking for because it no longer existed. "Would you like to hear something, son?"

I smiled back at him and said yes.

He started singing in a low, gravely voice that gradually rose, "There's a great big beautiful tomorrow, a beautiful tomorrow, mmm, mmm…"

He pronounced the lyrics meticulously, sounding out each syllable, albeit with melody somewhat lacking. He sang seriously, without any trace of irony. When he finished, he gave me a proud smile and asked, seemingly in earnest, "How was that, Doc?"

I asked Mr. Sardone to have a seat in the waiting room so I could talk to his daughter, and he complied.

She explained that he had been showing signs of confusion and faltering memory for some time now, but this last event really frightened her and her mom. I said it was clear that her father was suffering a dementia, probably an Alzheimer's type given the insidious decline. I explained that it is typical in these conditions to have meticulous preservation of some of the most remote memories, such as his visit to the World's Fair many decades ago. We found humor in the fact that we had both visited the fairgrounds as very young children—the daughter was probably a few years older than me—but neither could recall the details that her father seemed to retain, including the lyrics of the song. I did, however, have a clear recollection of the tune and a definite but somewhat dim memory of the ride. It is still called the Carousel of Progress and to this day remains operational at Disney World.

That evening, in the quiet of my study, I did some detective work, nothing too elaborate. I consulted our collective memory on the global internet. This is what I learned. Progressland was one of the most popular pavilions of the 1964 World's Fair. General Electric commissioned Walt Disney to develop a show that reflected his fervent optimism about technology and humanity's future. The Disney Imagineers—as the creative engineering team was called then (and still is today)—created an audio-animatronics family, human-like robots that could talk and move with some degree of realism (the current Hall of Presidents at Disney World is another example), and renowned songwriters Richard and Robert Sherman wrote the original song recited by my patient earlier in my office. The basic plot depicts an animatronic family throughout the twentieth century with each scene centered on a seasonal holiday. With the exception of some minor changes over the years due to technological advances, such as video games, cell phones, and home computers, little has been changed since its original inception. Once seated, you can travel across each scene and witness the progress of technological changes with each era.

The first act illustrated the typical American family—a mom, dad, son, and daughter and occasional grandparents—at the turn of the twentieth century on Valentine's Day, extolling the virtues of the newfangled telephone and washing machine. The second era takes place around 1927 when the family could enjoy electric lighting and radio on the Fourth of July. In the third act, set around Halloween 1947, the family is watching television. The final act, set around Christmas, depicts the family playing a wide-screen virtual reality game of space travel while Dad uses voice-command kitchen appliances.

At Disney World's Tomorrowland it remains as a monument of gee-whiz optimism and hopeful futurism with a hint of nostalgia in our cynical age. Hearing Mr. Sardone recite the song reanimated my own memories of family trips to the Magic Kingdom, when my family was young and intact, and filled with boundless enthusiasm and infinite possibility, which, inevitably with time and experience, may be eroded but never extinguished.

The word "nostalgia" is derived from two Greek words meaning "homecoming" and "pain" or "ache." It implies a longing or being homesick for something good that was lost through the passage of time. Deep in the hippocampus-amygdala complexes—we have one on both sides of our temporal lobes—long-term memory storage and its emotional content is consolidated. Good memories and the bad ones too. In animals, fear conditioning is permanently encoded there. Mr. Sardone, in his lost and demented state, was grasping for a happy experience long ago that echoed through his mind like a cry through some decaying canyon.

The fading echoes reverberated through my mind as well, longing for a lost tomorrow.

The Palace in My Head

It has been said that in the end all we are left with are our memories, if we're lucky. Diabolical conditions like Alzheimer's, traumatic brain injury, and stroke can rob from us the last precious remnants of our former lives. Each of us carries around, in the confines of our head, the memories of our unique and unrepeatable experiences complete with our own themes, narrative arcs, tragedies, and joys. Each brain has a hundred billion neurons and a hundred trillion stories.

Memories aren't only visual, although our primary recollections are often seen through the mind's eye as we imagine a past scene or event. However, we not only see memories, but we also smell, taste, and hear them through the magic of incredibly complex neural circuitry. The painful cry of a hurt child (especially one of your own) can be permanently encoded in your auditory cortex just as the face of that child is embedded in your brain's visual cortex. The sounds and visions of our past may haunt or delight us, and they are mostly with us until we die.

Elderly and widowed, but still independent, Mrs. Locasto lived alone. Although rather elegant and articulate, she was a lonely woman. Her two daughters, married with their own families, lived out of state and across the country. She was estranged from one of her daughters—a family inheritance issue or some such matter—and so Mrs. L. rarely saw her teenage grandchildren and was closer with her other daughter, but she never could make the trip to Chicago where they lived.

For many years Mrs. L. had suffered epilepsy. Her episodes were not the typical dramatic fall to the ground, convulsing unconsciously with limbs flailing, kind. She would stop suddenly in midsentence or midtask and stare blankly into space. After a minute or so, she would come back, a little dazed and sometimes a little embarrassed if in the company of others. Sometimes people with epilepsy experience those little warnings, premonitions, or auras just before the dreaded seizure. Mrs. L. denied any auras or warnings prior to her staring spells. She would take medication to prevent, or at least reduce, the occurrence of these episodes. She seemed to be very reliable and compliant regarding her treatment, which is why I was continuously perplexed by her recurrent seizures. She had taken the same drug, carbamezapine, for many years with generally good results and tolerance.

I was called to the local ER one night to evaluate her. She had some friends over and was preparing a spaghetti dinner when she became unresponsive and stared blankly while standing in her kitchen. She collapsed and hit her head on a table top. Terribly frightened, her guests called 911 and an ambulance rushed her to the hospital. An emergency CAT scan of her brain proved to be normal. There was no contusion or bleeding from the head trauma, but she did suffer a superficial scalp laceration which the ER doctor sutured. I met her there, and she seemed embarrassed over the whole incident. I recommended increasing her seizure medication dosage a little and sent her home.

On subsequent visits to the office she seemed to be doing well. She said she was tolerating her medication and seemed to have good compliance—medical jargon meaning she took it reliably. She was a little upset regarding my advice not to drive her car for now, but this is standard advice for someone who has suffered a recent seizure. Driving can pose major risks if a person suddenly loses consciousness.

Early one morning, several weeks later, the ER called to let me know that once again Mrs. L. had been seen there and was being admitted. She had collapsed just outside her home, and a neighbor spotted her lying on the front porch. In the ER she stared and blinked repetitively and did not respond, nor did she show any signs of being consciously aware. This kind of clinical situation can generally be life-threatening. Recurrent seizures—whether the convulsive kind (where the body shakes uncontrollably) or, as in this case, the nonconvulsive kind (where a person enters a kind of trancelike state, referred to as complex-partial epilepsy)—can be life-threatening and may result in permanent brain damage, respiratory failure, coma, and death. In this case of near status epilepticus (or recurrent uncontrolled seizing), her seizures broke before any permanent damage occurred with the administration of some intravenous seizure medicine, including lorezapam (a pharmacological cousin of Valium). She was admitted for observation overnight and was advised to see me in the next day or so.

A couple of days later, Mrs. L. presented to my office. She was particularly somber, and this was somewhat unusual for her as she often tried to be cheerful. She became tearful as I brought up a discussion about her recent hospitalization. It was clear that she was remorseful over her poor seizure control and blamed herself. She was very apologetic.

"I'm just so sorry over all the trouble I've caused. I'm so ashamed, you know. I didn't mean to put you and the hospital staff through so much trouble," she whispered. "I have to tell you something, something I've been doing or rather not doing that I didn't tell the ER docs."

"What is it, Mrs. Locasto?" I was somewhat intrigued and had no idea what dark secret she was about to reveal to me.

"You know my seizure medicine; I'm supposed to take it every day." I nodded. "Well, I often skip a day or two sometimes. I've learned over the years that my seizures are very sensitive to missing a dose or two. I'll always have an aura or two if I miss just a dose or so. I guess my brain is sensitive to even a slight drop in the drug level."

"That's right, when your carbamezapine level declines, your seizure threshold drops, and you have the potential for more auras and seizures. I think that's why you had those multiple seizures recently. Your carbamezapine blood level was a little low; that's why your dosage was increased in the ER, and we'll continue that for now. Hopefully this won't happen again."

"But, Doctor, you don't understand; I've been deliberately skipping dosages. I have to, you know."

Now I was somewhat perplexed. Medication compliance can be a big issue, especially in the older population. Some of the elderly patients can't afford the high cost of the multiple drugs they need to take on a daily basis, but I knew this was not the problem with Mrs. L. She was meticulous in nature as well, so I knew that she wasn't forgetful or irresponsible.

"Why have you been skipping dosages?" I asked plainly.

"You know I have those auras sometimes when I just get that sick feeling in the pit of my stomach, just before I have one of my staring spells."

I nodded, "Yes, that's quite typical." These prodromal symptoms arise from deep within the temporal lobes; we call them gustatory auras. They originate from the same place in the brain where the sensation of déjà vu, religious awe, and that anxious, butterflies-in-the-stomach feeling begin.

"Well, I have other auras too, different ones that in the past few years will often precede a seizure. I will hear the voices of my grandchildren, at least as I recall their voices when they were younger and I would see them regularly. They are as clear as day, talking about a bike ride or baking cookies in my kitchen—you know, remembrances of things we did years ago. It's all very vivid. It'll happen just before a seizure. Now I realized that when I take the medication regularly, it stops the episodes.

They never happen. I've learned to kind of look forward to them, even if it means having a seizure or two. When it happens, it's all so real, more than just a memory, like watching a home movie, but I really *feel* it." Her eyes watered, and so did mine a little.

I did the dutiful thing as a neurologist. I explained how dangerous it could be for her to continue to skip dosages of her carbamezapine. I explained how she already had ended up in the ER, how status epilepticus, convulsive or nonconvulsive (her type), could be life-threatening and cause permanent brain damage. I suggested perhaps referring her to a psychologist or psychiatrist to consider treatment for depression. I didn't expect her to follow any of this advice. She had found a way to capture a few evanescent moments of joy in her lonely life. The cost was high. She would have to suffer seizures—staring spells where she became unconscious, drooled, and sometimes urinated on herself. As long as no one knew, she wouldn't be embarrassed. She was a proud woman, and I now understood why she was so mortified by the ER visits. But for her it was worth it. She could conjure up lost memories, joyous ones. She could hear the voices of her grandchildren like echoes reverberating from deep within her temporal lobes, the hippocampus formations that store all our precious memories, many of them long forgotten.

"There's a palace in my head," she finally said to me. "The children play in it. Sometimes I can see them and hear them too…there's a palace in my head."

The Monster Within

There are many kinds of monsters, real and imagined, natural and supernatural, fictional and real. Odysseus was tormented by the beautiful but deadly Sirens. Dante descended into the dark depths of hell and witnessed humans transformed into hideous monsters as punishment for their earthly sins. As a child I was enthralled by the British Hammer Horror film series, Technicolor re-creations of the classic Frankenstein and Dracula movies. Monsters can be part of the natural world—terrorists, serial killers, and tyrants like Hitler. Otherworldly monsters, such as vampires and zombies, are thought to represent subconscious fears that we carry with us. Still, some beasts are sprung from our very own fabric, our character, and our minds.

I opened up a standard psychiatric handbook and read a specific passage quietly to the mother of seventeen-year-old Logan while he sat in the waiting room. Tall and gangly, with an explosion of blond-brown hair, he waited quietly. My office secretary would later note to me that he never seemed to blink and stared at his feet, never glancing at the TV or the pile of magazines next to him.

"Mrs. Gill, I want you to listen carefully to this," and I began, paraphrasing where necessary to avoid some of the textbook technical jargon.

> The disorder referred to as schizophrenia is characterized by abnormalities in the content and form of thought, abnormalities in sensory experience, and a dilapidation over time in social and interpersonal functioning. The abnormalities in the content of thought that are common in schizophrenia are delusions and first-rank symptoms such as thought broadcasting and thought insertion, somatic hallucinations, auditory hallucinations and feelings of actions controlled by outside forces, and delusional perceptions (e.g., the perception that one's thoughts are being read, taken, or inserted by an outside agent). Delusions of grandeur or persecution are common…
>
> Thought disorder as manifested through speech is typically present. Ideas that are entirely unrelated are believed to be causally connected as exhibited in the sentence "The sky is blue so I will go to the bank," where the ideas might be connected in the patient's mind because the bank building looks blue.

Auditory hallucinations are experienced as criticisms or commands in the third person, often from multiple voices, such as "Look at her brush her teeth; I'll bet she is going to get sick."

Changes in thinking include inability to follow a train of thought, seeing or hearing things that aren't real, and paranoia. Changes in emotions include moodiness and irritability, and being fearful. Changes in behavior can include talking to him- or herself, the inability to make or keep friends with social withdrawal and increasing social isolation, poor personal hygiene, inappropriate emotional responses and behavior…

Schizophrenia-like disorders can be seen in association with several neurological illnesses, including structural brain disease.

The last sentence was the one that heralded desperate hope.

"They asked me to bring my son to you. They said we have to rule out any neurological problems that could be causing some issues. He's not crazy, and I won't accept that as an explanation. He's a bright young man; he plays three musical instruments and has a real aptitude for math. Logan's not crazy…he's not…" Her voice cracked.

This was a mother defending her son. She was angry over what was happening and terrified even more. I remember she was meticulously groomed. She may have felt that her life and her son's life were unraveling, but she was determined not to have her appearance divulge that story.

"He's had every type of blood test. They checked out his thyroid three times. I know hyperthyroidism can cause delirium and psychosis. I had them check his cortisol levels too, and they did a heavy metal urine screen. Are there other toxins that they should look for? PCBs, Thimersol, BPAs…there are so many. I have a printout from the EPA I got online. And there are molds, fungus that are carcinogenic. I had the house checked for radon too. It's a turn-of-the-century Victorian, so who knows, it's so old."

I wanted to interrupt her, but she was trying to get out as much as possible while holding back the tears. Her son was sitting in my waiting room. I had not yet met him. My concerned secretary would also later tell me that during the entire time he appeared to be mumbling to the rhododendron plant.

"Mrs. Gill…" I tried to speak very gently, attempting to counterbalance her barely controlled frenzy. "I know that Logan's internist and psychiatrist referred him to me for further evaluation, but let's start at the beginning, okay?"

She took an audible sigh and spoke in a hushed tone. "Logan's a good boy. He was always a good student, played soccer. He can play the flute and violin. He's always been quiet and studious."

"That's good, Mrs. Gill. How's everything at home? Do you have any other children?"

"No, my husband and I tried but we had fertility issues, so we were grateful and surprised when I got pregnant with

Logan. We've lived in the same house since he was born, same school, no major changes at all."

"When did the trouble start?" I asked, trying to get to heart of the matter at hand.

"I guess around his sophomore year in high school. He gave up soccer because he said it was taking too much of his time—he was already taking some advanced placement and honors courses. He started spending more and more time in his room. We really didn't think anything strange about that because he was doing well academically. He started drifting away from his friends. There were a lot of little things, looking back, that we started to notice. He would skip a day or two and not shower. He got very fussy about food. One of his favorites is my baked macaroni and cheese, but one day, when I made it for dinner, he said it looked disgusting. I think he said it 'looked like animal guts,' and he never ate it again."

Her cell phone rang and she put it on silent mode. She continued, "I thought to myself that so far this could just be normal teenager angst, academic pressure, social changes of high school, nothing really outstanding here.

"One day, the school called me. They said some students found him on the bathroom floor talking to himself; he seemed very upset. They asked me to bring him home."

"What happened? Did someone upset him?" I asked.

"No, he said the bathroom was disgusting, full of germs, and that his history teacher knew that and knew that this would upset him…I don't know, he was very confused. I took him home, and he quieted down. I don't think anything really happened."

One day, he came home from school inconsolable. He cried to his mother, "Mommy, why do they keep calling me stupid and worthless, why, why? Why do they keep telling me I'm a 'fatal error'?" His mother was prepared to march into school and ferret out the callous classmates who were tormenting her son until Logan screamed at his mom that the "voices were all inside, every night especially when it's quiet or I'm alone. They curse at me, yell at me!"

"I was terrified," Mrs. Gill explained, "and that's when I asked my husband to return early from his business trip. We both took him to a psychiatrist that our family internist recommended."

She took a deliberate breath, paused, and then continued, "He says it's probably a psychiatric disorder…He, well, he says we have to rule out any neurological condition, but that it could be a schizophrenia type of condition. He's hearing voices, imagining things; he's becoming reclusive…it's so horrible. He says there's medication, but he wants to make sure first that there's no other possible cause." She began sobbing again. Her son seemed to be descending into madness before her very eyes.

"Has he become violent or tried to make any indication that he wants to hurt himself?" I asked delicately, really inquiring about any homicidal or suicidal ideation.

"No, not at all. But he knows something is wrong with him, at least sometimes. And then sometimes he just doesn't have a clue. The other day he spent an hour scrubbing down the bathroom floor before he took a shower. My house is spotless, but he said it felt dirty...I caught him on his hands and knees using a Brillo pad; he was muttering to himself about keeping everything clean. He practically destroyed the marble floor."

Finally, I called Logan into the exam room. He was polite, quiet, and a little nervous. His somber demeanor gave no indication of the maelstrom that was brewing inside his head. I performed a perfunctory neurological exam. There was no family history of any neurological or psychiatric conditions, such as Huntington's disease and other conditions that can sometimes mimic mental illness. There was no history of drug or alcohol abuse, already confirmed by his blood and urine tests. I asked him if he was as concerned about what was happening as his parents were.

"Yeah, I mean I guess so, but it's not such a big deal. They worry a lot."

I asked him about hearing disembodied voices talking to him, scolding him.

"Yeah, sometimes." He shrugged his shoulders without volunteering more.

"All right, I'm going to send you for some routine studies—a brain MRI, electroencephalogram, and a few blood tests. Is that okay with you?"

He nodded yes and within a week the studies were complete. As expected, everything was completely normal. Brain MRI revealed no suspicious tumors, electroencephalogram showed no abnormal brain wave activity, and blood serology, including repeat drug screens for amphetamines, barbiturates, opiates, cannabis, etc., were all negative. I explained this to Logan's mom in the office.

"Don't tell me everything is normal, Dr. Adamo. With all due respect, nothing is normal!" She was obviously angry at what I thought would be welcome news. "I'm taking him to a university hospital. I know they can do more in-depth testing there," she said indignantly.

I agreed halfheartedly, so as not to upset her, and provided her with some names of neurologists at the nearby academic medical center.

Weeks later, Logan and his mom returned armed with cerebral PET and SPECT scan reports, functional MRI brain-imaging results, and second and third opinions from an Ivy League medical center. The studies revealed, once again, no evidence of a brain tumor, encephalitis, hydrocephalus, multiple sclerosis, Parkinson's disease, Huntington's disease, or adrenoleukodystrophy, to name just a few of the diseases and disorders that Mrs. Gill was convinced her son might be afflicted with. She seemed more frustrated than ever.

"Look, Mrs. Gill, there should be some degree of relief. Logan is not suffering a fatal neurological disorder, and there is hope with medication and counseling for schizophrenia disorders." I tried to be optimistic, realizing how devastating a chronic diagnosis like schizophrenia can be. It is a major cause of chronic disability, and treatment with potent antipsychotic drugs can be variably successful and fraught with miserable side effects. I used my standby example of John Nash, the Nobel Prize-winning economist who struggled with schizophrenia his entire life. But she knew all this, at least on an intellectual level, and was grappling with something else.

"There has to be an explanation for this," she fired back. "There is no family history of mental illness, he had a normal childhood, and we were good parents, loving parents. He's being swallowed up by this…his personality, his school performance, everything is falling apart…maybe he needs a brain biopsy. Then they can see what's wrong; they could examine the pathology directly!"

I started to realize where this was headed. A tidy diagnosis, such as a brain tumor, would be far more comprehensible, and in some ways, if not fatal, even more treatable. We could identify the problem, cut it out physically, and return her son intact. This disease was eroding his character. I took out a psychiatry text from my training and read it to her. It wasn't until I read the very last sentence to her that I realized exactly what she was grappling with:

Schizophrenia-like disorders can be seen in association with several neurological disorders, including structural brain disease.

It was clear to me now. I smiled at her. She was holding back the tears. Logan sat mute; he seemed mercifully unaware of his mother's turmoil.

"I know you want there to be a neat and clean diagnosis here, something fixable like a brain tumor that can be cut out and removed, but keep in mind that schizophrenia is treatable and not lethal like brain tumors can be." I was trying to be optimistic but fully understood what a terrible disease we were dealing with. Schizophrenia erodes one's personality and character. I think even Logan recognized this behind his blank expression.

For the next six months, Logan and his mother took a whirlwind tour of alternative medicine. They visited an acupuncturist, energy field specialist (I never figured out what that is, and Logan wasn't sure either), a homeopath who rubbed his scalp with a diluted solution of wolfsbane (a flower), and a chiropractor who "redirected his spinal energies" (it gave Logan a headache).

He was finally seen by a psychiatrist and psychologist at the local university hospital, started a regimen of neuroleptic and mood-stabilizing drugs, and began showing some promising improvement.

On their last visit to see me, Logan seemed more astute. In the waiting room, he read a magazine and ignored the rhododendron plant. His mom, still misty-eyed when she spoke of him but smiling, said he was on track to graduate on time and was likely to be accepted to one of the local universities so he could commute and not interrupt his psychiatric care.

Before leaving she confided in me, "I feel like we at least have a piece of our son back, but I wouldn't wish this upon anyone."

The Banquet

It has been said throughout the ages that the driving force of civilization, including science, medicine, and culture, is the quest to prevent death, to live forever. Throughout history, science has sought to make life better with the always unrealized hope of eradicating death. Religion offers the hope of eternal life, whether it is the Judeo-Christian heaven or the Buddhist nirvana. We humans are capable of such majestic achievements that allow us to transcend the limits nature has imposed upon us. A piece of each of us lives on in our work, in our children, and in the memories of our loved ones. Nonetheless, it would seem that we are ultimately doomed to return to the earth from which we sprang and vanish forever. Most us carry on with this haunting realization and try to find daily fulfillment in our lives, our families, and the many joys of just being alive. But there is sometimes a thin line between the sensible recognition that the clock is ticking and the relentless fear of our mortality.

Jerry sat quietly in the trauma room. He had just crashed his vintage 1977 Chevrolet Monte Carlo into a towering oak across from his home in what seemed to be a feeble suicide attempt. His wife, Alice, heard the crash of what was previously a well-cared-for coup wedged against the immovable tree, the front hood buckled in an upside-down V-shape. She screamed out his name and called 911.

His physical injuries were minor, some scratches and bruises and a mild concussion.

Psychiatry was called to the ER because the patient readily admitted that the car accident was a deliberate suicide attempt. I was called, as is typical in these kinds of cases, because there was concern regarding head trauma and a possible seizure. The astute nurse informed me, "Brain CT is normal, and he remembers the entire accident, so it doesn't sound like he had a seizure either before or after the crash. But the guy's a bit of an oddball, really evasive and really somber. Maybe he's just embarrassed."

Jerry was in his midthirties; both he and his wife were white-collar professionals. Together for over a decade, the marriage, by design or chance, was childless. He had been treated in the past with antidepressant meds for mild depression. He worked at the same financial firm for nearly eight years and had advanced to an upper-level position. He had no major medical problems and did not abuse alcohol or drugs. The psychiatry resident on call warned me that he was very despondent and would be admitted for close observation and one-on-one observation due to the high suicide risk.

As I examined him, he seemed to be very cooperative, as well as apologetic about the entire "incident" as he called it.

"I'm so sorry about this; I feel so ashamed. All you doctors are so professional, but what's the point?"

"The point is for you not to die." I smiled at him. "You're a young guy with what seems to be a good life. Why did you try to hurt yourself?"

He stared directly ahead at the tiled wall but seemed to be focusing on something beyond it. He answered slowly, "I've realized for a long time now…that, well, I'm virtually dead. I know my liver and heart have already rotted. My brain is just melting away; I know it is. I know it sounds crazy, but it's how I feel. I don't want Alice to deal with this; she shouldn't have to…so I decided to just end it. Unsuccessfully, I guess."

I quickly responded, hoping that my medical logic would provide him with insight. "All your tests including brain scan and labs are normal. It doesn't look like you sustained any serious injuries at all. You're not dying!"

"Doctor, you don't get it. I may be already dead; I don't know. We're all doomed anyway. We're all going back in the ground; we're all just a banquet for the flowers and the worms and the soil. I think the worms are already inside of me, eating away until I just vanish, vanish into nothing…"

At this point I didn't know what to make of Jerry. Was he speaking in metaphors and was really just a depressed man with a morbid preoccupation? Was he psychotic, harboring bizarre delusions completely divorced from reality? Was he a phony, a malingerer craving attention or permanent disability benefits?

In the days that followed, I visited Jerry in the hospital for routine post-concussion evaluations. A follow-up brain MRI proved normal as were his urine and serum toxicology screens for any illicit drug use or overdose.

He was placed on an antidepressant (Lexapro) and a mood stabilizer (Gabapentin, originally a seizure and nerve pain medication that doubles as a psychiatric drug for depression-related mood swings and bipolar disorder), but improvement was not expected to occur in the immediate future. He was still on suicide observation, so he could not yet be discharged. His presence in the hospital gave each of his consulting doctors—the internist, cardiologist, and gastroenterologist—the opportunity to investigate his myriad complaints from chest pain to abdominal pain to groin pain. Nothing turned up on his multiple blood tests, MRIs, echocardiograms, endoscopies, and even a skin biopsy. He soon gained the reputation as an annoying hypochondriac. He remained convinced, despite the abundance of medical evidence against his fixed belief, that he was rapidly dying and "rotting like an old tree stump in the woods, a real banquet," as he would often utter to the hospital staff. His wife remained dedicated but perplexed, having known him to be a bit of a depressive type but never to this extent.

Throughout this ordeal Jerry remained emotionally detached. To the casual observer, he may have appeared stoic in the face of his imagined fatal illness, but this was something different. The psychiatrists call it "derealization," a certain disconnection from reality where a person feels emotionally isolated from what should be a harrowing experience. Somehow the neural connections between the rational prefrontal lobes and the emotional amygdalae get frayed, resulting in a cold and detached view of one's imagined suffering.

As the week went by, there was no obvious improvement in Jerry's demeanor. He became increasingly despondent with persistent ruminations about death, dying, and the decaying of a seemingly healthy body. He told the cardiologist that he felt as if "insect larvae were growing inside my heart" and warned the gastroenterologist that "there's something rotting in my bowels," despite having recently undergone a normal colonoscopy. Yet, in every other way, he was rational and coherent.

When asked about the possibility of suicide, Jerry would answer, "I'm really already dead so suicide would serve no purpose." It took some time for his doctors to realize that he wasn't speaking metaphorically. He literally meant that he was either dead or very near death.

After two weeks of this, frustrated over his continued depression, psychiatry decided to shock him back to life.

Electroconvulsive therapy (ECT) involves sedating a patient under light general anesthesia and administering a jolt of electricity via two applied electrodes to the scalp. A generalized convulsion or seizure will result, lasting a few minutes, and gradually the patient will regain full consciousness. Despite our very limited understanding of how this seemingly rather violent procedure works, it is clear that its efficacy is undeniable. It is often used as a treatment of last resort in severely depressed patients because it will allow a rapid but temporary improvement. In conjunction with medication and therapy, a patient can steadily regain normal behavior.

Jerry was jolted with 150 volts; he seized and vomited, and after a couple of days was doing much better. He was totally mystified at how utterly obsessed with death he had become and seemed mortified over his past behavior. He was discharged to home and scheduled for close psychiatric follow-up.

"Was this just a case of really bad depression?" I asked the psychiatrist.

"Actually," he said, smiling, "I think this was a case of a rare disorder called Cotard's syndrome, and a relatively mild one at that. In more severe cases, a patient can be convinced that they are literally dead or have become walking zombies. Sometimes they even have psychotic delusions that they no longer exist."

Over the years Jerry would sometimes be referred back to me for relatively minor neurological issues (dizziness from an inner ear infection or an occasional migraine). He would always conclude his office visit with the following admonition:

"Keep your head up, enjoy the day, but never forget the banquet!"

Primun Non Nocere

The universal guiding principle of all physicians is embodied in the golden axiom "First, do no harm." It is both an exhortation and a warning. Philosophers call it by another, more technical name: nonmalificence. It means whatever you do, don't make things worse. Sometimes doing nothing in medicine is better than doing something. A situation may best be treated with reservation, not action, and the wisdom to know the difference. But sometimes doing nothing results from a failure of imagination, not considering all possibilities, or a missed or misdiagnosis. Sometimes doing nothing is worse.

The nurse wore a clean, crisp white uniform. I explained to her that I was referred to consult on one of the patients recently admitted to the nursing home. She pointed the way to a brightly lit sunroom at the end of the corridor. The "solarium," as it was referred to by the staff, was the only room in the complex that had more than one window. In fact, three of the four walls were glass, offering an unobstructed view of a small patch of woods, the ocean bay on the right, and the visitor parking lot on the left. The humble view seemed to encompass all of creation—the man-made concrete car lot, the untrammeled woods, the vast sea with sun and infinite sky. It was all here at the end of corridor 2C. And so was patient R. A., or Renee, as I would learn to call her.

The room was large and populated with an odd combination of hospital and civilian-type furniture—Formica tables with folding chairs, flimsy waiting room-type sofas, and hefty recliners, the latter probably donated from someone's home. An old Sony TV was in the corner. Van Gogh and Monet reproductions hung on the white walls, bleached by the constant sunlight exposure. Beneath the washed-out sunflowers sat Renee in a wheelchair, half covered with a yellow crocheted blanket. She was thirty-six, according to her chart, but looked older despite the long brown hair. Frail and tiny in stature, she spoke in a perpetual whisper.

She had been in the nursing home for about two months. There were concerns about her going home to her busy household of two teenage children and a husband. Her walking was still unsteady, and she was having some cognitive and memory difficulties as well. She persevered with physical therapy every day. Once athletic and strong, she had participated in a cross-country just a year ago.

"You're Dr. Adamo?" she asked meekly.

"Yes, the house physician called my office and asked me

to see you. We might be able to make some adjustments to your medication regimen. I think we can wean you off the anti-seizure and steroid meds. But first, if you don't mind, I'll need to take a few moments and review your chart. It's a pretty thick one." I smiled and looked down toward the ponderous volume.

"Yeah, a lot has happened in the past few months." She faintly smiled back.

I delved into the chart.

About four months ago, Renee visited her family doctor, something this once healthy young woman rarely needed to do. She had developed headaches. At first, they were a minor nuisance but they progressed. Occurring intermittently, they could be severe with throbbing and nausea. She found herself taking Motrin or Tylenol sometimes on a daily basis for over a month or two to get through her busy days until she finally relented and saw her family doctor. He promptly diagnosed her with migraines as she fit the age group, and her headaches shared some of the characteristics of this common disorder. Over the next two months or so, he prescribed a variety of popular migraine drugs, none of which worked well. The headaches persisted with no obvious explanation. Blood tests were normal as was an eye exam. So sure of the diagnosis despite the failure of medications to alleviate the pain, no brain MRI or CT was ordered. During one particularly severe episode, Renee's husband drove her to the local hospital ER. She was hurriedly prescribed some narcotic pain meds, Tylenol with codeine, by a busy staff doctor and swiftly sent home. The note read "36-year-old female with history of migraine presents with typical migraine."

She relied on that prescription for another week or two, but the headaches became more refractory.

One evening, while enjoying a school play, she noticed double images of all the stage players. Her family doctor finally referred her to a neurologist the next morning, and she promptly underwent a brain MRI, now over four months after her initial symptoms. It revealed a large right-hemisphere mass with swelling, a probable tumor.

"So it was double vision that finally convinced your doctor that something bad was happening?" I asked her, hoping to engage her in some conversation as we both had been quiet for several minutes.

She spoke slowly, with strained effort, a residual of the brain surgery. "It was a spring play, *The Sound of Music*. My daughter played…Liesl Von Trapp, you know, the oldest of the…Von Trapp children. I knew…once…the double vision started that my…headaches…couldn't be just migraine like… my doctor was telling me. I knew…something was going on, from day…one really."

I read on, fumbling through the thick volume, the binder almost bursting. At this point Renee was quickly sent to a neurosurgeon and was scheduled for a craniotomy to biopsy and remove as much of the mass as possible. Judging from the notes, there was still doubt on what the mass exactly was, but the doctors were sure that it had to be removed. It was growing dangerously bigger, increasing the intracranial pressure as evidenced by the severe headaches and visual loss. The notes also documented left arm and leg weakness developing at this point.

The craniotomy and tumor resection went well or "uneventful" as the progress notes described. Her speech was largely spared, but the hemiparesis (weakness of her left arm and leg) remained post-op.

The biopsy results ultimately yielded a definitive diagnosis. The mass was not a tumor but an abscess. It was puss filled and teaming with Staphylococcus aureus bacteria. It was speculated that a simple skin infection, perhaps a carbuncle or acne "zit," may have spilled a few bacteria into the bloodstream, which seeded in the brain. Not common but certainly not unheard of.

Renee looked down at the chart. It was opened to the postoperative report, which summarized the brain surgery she underwent.

"They told me I'm lucky…it was a brain abscess…not…a…tumor." She smiled, her face crooked from the stroke injury. She continued with effort in that staccato-like halting tone, "A tumor…would have been much worse. But my family…is…still upset. So…they…are suing." She looked down, as if ashamed to admit this to me.

She had survived but with complications: a stroke as well as speech and cognitive deficits that may never resolve. There was certainly a delay in diagnosis. A brain-imaging study, CT or MRI, should have been done months earlier in this young woman with unexplained, new onset headaches rather than assuming she suffered the relatively benign condition of migraine. The brain infection could have been detected early on before an abscess formed. Perhaps it could have been averted with antibiotics before it took form as a puss-filled sphere inside her head. And maybe these complications could have been completely avoided. The error here was in doing nothing rather than doing something wrong. Renee was now mostly wheelchair bound and no longer the active suburban mom she once prided herself on being.

Over the ensuing months there would be a lawsuit and finally a hefty settlement. There was a crime of sorts: misdiagnosis. There were perpetrators: an aged and kindly physician who misled himself into not considering the more serious diagnosis. There was the young and harried ER physician. And finally, there was Renee, the patient-victim.

We discussed some routine medical matters, such as medication adjustments. When it came time to leave, she smiled at me, turned toward the window, and looked resolutely at the immense ocean view before us.

"I'm… going to walk again, on…my…own. Maybe…not…run in the marathons…but I'll walk again. I know I will."

Of Minds and Maps*

The history of neurology can be viewed as the history of creating maps. In the nineteenth century, phrenologists tried to explain personality traits by developing a topography of cranial bumps. This now-debunked idea paved the way for an important neurologic tenet: the localization and specification of brain function. Paul Broca and Carl Wernicke, over a century and a half ago, used this principle to map out the mind, showing that the unique human ability of language is grounded in specific physical structures of the brain. This began a kind of Copernican revolution in the study of the brain and mind. We could finally begin to view the mind as a manifestation of the inner physical machinations of the brain and not some mysterious Cartesian "ghost in the machine."

As a neurology resident, I remember being told the classic aphorism "God must be a cartographer, for the brain is full of maps" by a pensive, gray-haired neuropathologist. He was not making a theological proclamation but a scientific point.

Retinotopic maps guide the visual cortex, tonotopic maps are found in Heschl's gyrus of the auditory cortex, and somatotopic homunculi inhabit our motor and sensory cortices. Confronted with the intimidating task of slicing and dicing this three-pound enigma in the neuropathology laboratory, it was reassuring to have map and atlas in hand.

Like the ancient ritual of trepination, we would cut out bone flaps to remove the glistening matter. Under the harsh fluorescent laboratory lights, the oozing brain fluid seemed luminous. Many of the brains we dissected had belonged to walking and talking people just days before the autopsies, sad victims of suddenly ruptured cerebral aneurysms and unexpected cardiac arrests. Holding a fresh human brain in your hands that just a few days ago was thinking and feeling, one cannot help but be astonished over the fact that a hundred billion jelly-like neurons with their hundred trillion connections somehow manage to create memory, emotion, language, a sense of personal identity, and, most mysterious of all, consciousness.

Ultimately, a map is a metaphor constructed by the mind to explain itself. Aristotle viewed the mind as a tabula rasa upon which nature and experience write their story to create our picture of reality. Many centuries ago later, Sigmund Freud created a tripartite model of the mind, dividing it into unconscious, preconscious, and conscious levels. In the past half century, another triune model of the brain became popular, this one looking at the brain in terms of its evolutionary history and dividing it into a reptilian brain stem, limbic system, and neocortex.

More recently, technological models have prevailed, likening the CNS to the internet or the most ubiquitous model, the computer. In this modern view, the brain is supposed to be a glorified Turing machine, processing information according to computational rules and producing a mental simulation of the environment with which we interact. But our brains do not just record and manipulate data, they also imbue meaning into everything we see, hear, touch, and feel. All our models and metaphors are ultimately impoverished because they can only vaguely signify the enormous complexities of the brain.

Like every student of the brain, I have spent countless hours memorizing and learning maps of the cerebral cortex, interconnections of the basal ganglia, neurotransmitter pathways, and the myriad anatomic tracts that span the brain like so much gossamer. The most memorable map of all, however, was one that was held up to my face one midnight by a desperate mother, who was almost too grief stricken to speak.

It was a bright autumn morning when this mother's daughter, Mary, was walking to school with two of her friends. All three were seniors in high school, and perhaps their conversation centered on topics like the upcoming senior prom, college acceptance letters, and boyfriends. As the girls crossed the street to their school, Mary was struck by a speeding van, her body sent hurling six feet into the air and crashing down on the hard pavement, her friends screaming in horror. She was hit with such momentum that her school backpack was later found three blocks away.

I first saw Mary in the bright fluorescent dayglow of the intensive care unit. With a brain full of blood, she was in a deep coma on a mechanical respirator. As the days passed, it became clear that Mary could only muster the most primitive brain stem reflexes.

Her mother kept a constant bedside vigil. One evening, clearly exasperated over some minor nursing care issue, she approached me with a book in hand. "Where is my daughter's mind?" she angrily asked, opening her book in front of me. The thick volume appeared to be a college neuroscience textbook. She opened it up and turned to a page containing colorful diagrams of the brain in cross section. She gestured toward the pictures. "Does she have any memory, does she feel any sadness, does she know I'm here with her?" These questions were not philosophical ruminations but rather a mother's desperate attempt to comprehend the enormity of this unbearable tragedy.

I gently closed the textbook. "You must understand," I whispered. "The damage is pervasive; the brain and brain stem have suffered irreversible injury."

"But what about the thalamus and the reticular activating system? I've read that they're very important for the consciousness," she whispered back to me.

Her question, I think, was rhetorical. She knew that the answer she was looking for could not be found in the esoteric language of neurology.

Her somber question "Where is my daughter's mind?"

echoed in my mind during the drive back home that night. Do we have any brain maps that can identify where consciousness, self-awareness, or the elusive "I" that narrates our personal history can be found? Not yet. There is no single master control center that mediates consciousness or the self. When it comes to language and memory, this problem may not be as intractable. We know that written and spoken language ability is lateralized in a dominant hemisphere for all humans. Language is a product of several distinct and interconnected areas of the brain, and we know that the temporal lobes and hippocampi are crucial for memory storage. Indeed, we now have intricate maps elucidating both structure and function, derived from elaborate imaging studies. But there is no telltale glow on a functional MRI that divulges the presence of a center that harbors consciousness or personality identity.

So where does the mind go when the brain is destroyed? Religion has always upheld the idea of an eternal and immutable soul, and perhaps this idea comforted Mary's mother. But such solace cannot be provided by neurology, where consciousness and the self must be explained, if ever, in the lexicon of science.

By the time I arrived home that evening, Mary had suffered her second and final cardiac arrest. I thought that somehow I should have been more eloquent, more empathetic, in this tragic circumstance. Without turning to religious symbolism, however, the best I could ponder was this. Mary now exists only as an encoded memory deep in the brains of her loved ones, a kind of virtual reality figment that can be played over and over again. But of Mary's mind, it is lost forever. Of course, I could not bear to say this to Mary's mom, but I really did not need to. With the neurology textbook in hand, she realized, as I did, that some of our most detailed and precise maps are woefully inadequate.

* Originally published in *Neurology*, April 14, 2009, vol.72 no.15.

The Carnival*

When I was a young boy, my parents took me to a traveling country carnival in Upstate New York where my grandparents lived. In the days before children became mesmerized by the hypnotic glow of the video screen, the country fair was a major form of public entertainment. The Ferris wheels and roller coasters offered the promise of experiencing such exciting and frightening neurological symptoms as acute vertigo and disequilibrium, along with the occasional unintended nausea and vomiting. As twilight approached on that summer evening, my parents and I wandered to the darkened periphery of the fairground, away from the buzzing noises and bright lights. We slowly approached a small rectangular tent with a pitched rooftop. A string of incandescent light bulbs softly illuminated the flimsy structure. I clearly remember the small sign (or warning) outside the doorway that stated "This Exhibit Not for Entertainment."

Once inside, my parents assumed a somber and almost

pious silence. The large rectangular room was very quiet, the walls lined with shelves that housed glass jars of various sizes. Each receptacle contained a fetus, some relatively normal looking, while others were so hideously deformed as to be unrecognizable as human. These pitiful creatures were in various stages of embryologic development. Some looked like normal-term babies, some looked like large tadpoles, some had enormous swollen heads, tails, extra arms or legs, or three eyes. Being a young science-fiction enthusiast, I wondered if any one of them might be an extraterrestrial from perhaps the red sands of Mars or the stormy world of Jupiter. It was clear to me that none of them were alive, and I thought that was certainly for the better. None of the jars were labeled, and no explanation as to the origin of these loathsome creatures was offered. As we walked down the corridors, my parents would whisper and shake their heads. It became clear to me that this house of horrors was really a very sad place. Although at this young age I certainly did not possess the vocabulary or the intellect to frame analytical questions about the human brain, I still wondered about what human abilities these poor creatures may have once possessed. Did these sad beings think and feel? Did they have memories and emotions? Did they once have conscious awareness and recognize their miserable plight? Their images left an indelible impression on a young mind and still haunt me to this day.

It would be over two decades before I would revisit this place in another form, a modern child neurology clinic at the university hospital where I was a young neurologist in training. It would be here that I would finally gain some scientific understanding and perhaps some human insight into what I gazed upon so long ago. The university hospital clinic functioned like a well-oiled machine at its best. Eager medical students, bright young resident physicians, and experienced attendings fervently discussed cases both common and unusual. Such an antiseptic academic environment, however, might not seem conducive to producing awe and wonder. Nevertheless, I would often experience this sense just anticipating my weekly visit to this clinic. To be sure, there would be plenty of routine cases at our weekly sessions: autistic toddlers, children with epilepsy, patients with neurogenetic disorders like neurofibromatosis. Once a month, however, we would see children with profoundly devastating neurological conditions, for whom no real treatment could be offered other than so-called supportive care. These tragic cases often prompted me to speculate about the human brain, consciousness, and memory. One particular case I vividly recall.

Megan was a bright and perky young mother of three children, the youngest of which she would bring to our clinic every few months. This male child would come wrapped in blankets in a stroller. His mother would lovingly describe his eating schedule and bathing habits to us. His clothes and blankets were decorated with Disney cartoon characters. As I examined him for the first time, I realized this was a large baby with a big head. His eyes stared intently or darted about chaotically. The limbs would adjust position in a seemingly voluntary manner, and I thought he cooed once or twice. As a young neurologist who was just starting to develop some self-confidence over my clinical skills, I was stunned when I learned that the baby was three and a half years old. Furthermore, this child had no brain. He was a terrible victim of an anencephalic-like syndrome. His head was mainly filled with fluid and a thin mantle of cerebral cortex. He could not think, learn, or remember in any real sense. He would never talk or walk. Most of what he did in life involved primitive brain stem reflexes. From what we know, no true self-awareness or capacity for memory or emotion could exist. I immediately recalled the denizens of that sad carnival long ago. I realized that those poor creatures were human anencephalics and hydrocephalics who were trapped in a zombie-like state. They could never have known consciousness, memory, or emotion, at least not in the way that you and I experience them.

Somewhere along the way I learned that the historical meaning of "carnival," at least as it was known in the Middle Ages, involves the celebration of the unity of the human race. No matter what our station or abilities in life, we are all mortal creatures who enter and exit the world with no choice in the matter. Life can be as painful as it is ephemeral, but it can also be joyous and wondrous. It is the tragedy and majesty of life that carnival tries to reconcile.

*Originally published in *Neurology*, July 22, 2008, vol.71 no. 4.

Lost in the Fugue

In music, a fugue refers to a composition that has a recurrent theme in several different voices. By way of musical analogy, each of our lives can be viewed similarly. We each have our own personal struggles, obstacles, and themes that may recur, in different variations, at various stages, as we move on in life. For most of us, the composition of our lives is a fairly continual narrative. Fortunately, very few of us will ever experience what is referred to as a "fugue state" (also referred to as a dissociative or psychogenic fugue). This enigmatic disorder—popularized in films like the Jason Bourne series and Hitchcock's classic *Spellbound*—is as mysterious as it is fascinating. I submit for your approval the case of Jane T.

"They told me I should see a neurologist after being discharged from the hospital, and they gave me your name," said Jane with her bright smile and youthful face.

"All right, do you know why, Jane? I'm still waiting for your hospital records to come over the fax," I responded.

"I think it's because I took an 'unscheduled vacation'," gesturing air quotes with her hands and smiling sarcastically.

"Well, that certainly doesn't sound like the kind of issue you'd need to see a neurologist for."

"No, it certainly isn't." She smiled again.

Five weeks ago, Jane, a high school English teacher in her late twenties, was following her usual routine: class every day, supervising the student newspaper, and lately weekends and evenings spent at the hospital. Her mother had recently received a bad diagnosis: her previously treated breast cancer had returned with a vengeance. There was metastasis to the liver, bone, and brain as well. Jane was an only child, the product of a loving home with parents who doted on her. And now her mother was dying. Medical complications prevented her from being discharged to hospice care, so she remained bed stricken in the ICU. Jane dutifully visited her every day or evening and watched her fiftyish mother slowly become more and more lethargic until one Saturday afternoon, with her daughter at her bedside, she closed her glassy eyes and never opened them again.

Jane returned to school after a brief hiatus of about a week. Dedicated to her students, and not yet encumbered by a family of her own, she was eager to return to work. She quickly seemed to get back to her routine: classes, tutoring, meetings. One rainy evening she booked a flight to a Caribbean island. It was easy. She had frequent-flyer miles, arranged for a same-day late flight online, and even got an Uber cab as part of the package deal. She grabbed her overcoat, purse, and passport, no suitcases, and was whisked off to the airport. In a few hours, her plane landed, and she wandered the sun-bleached streets of her paradise getaway.

Twilight approached and the flow of tourists in town ebbed. Jane, tired from her hurried exodus, found a quiet patch of shrubbery on the local beach, lay down, and fell asleep. She slept undisturbed most of that evening under the tropical starlight and woke up to a beautiful sunrise. She paid no attention to her disheveled appearance, found a public bathroom, freshened up a little, and resumed walking aimlessly, hoping that she was headed back to town. Nearby, some local police were not oblivious to the sight of this young, unkempt American clutching her purse and still wearing her raincoat. They approached her cautiously and convinced her to let them escort her to the local hospital.

Back at home, her father, older brother, and boyfriend were frantically trying to find where Jane had vanished to. It was unheard of for her to miss school with no warning. Dreaded thoughts of abduction, accident, and even suicide filled their worried heads.

At the Caribbean clinic, she underwent some blood tests, a drug screen, and even a brain CT, all of which were normal. Jane could not offer the doctors there any clear explanation for her behavior. She had not committed any violations or crimes, and so the police were happy to bring her to the airport for a return flight. Before leaving, she called her dad to let him know not to worry: "Hi, Dad, I'm on my way home. I'm here, um, I think Nassau, but I'll be on the next flight. The police and the doctors were very nice, um...see you soon."

Her family and boyfriend nervously waited for her plane to arrive and hurried her off to the hospital once her feet touched New York. Still seemingly bewildered, she asked, "But didn't I just come from there?"

In the local hospital ER, the medical ritual she had undergone a few hours ago in the Caribbean was repeated, only this time the more sophisticated American version was conducted. She underwent three different brain MRIs, an EEG, cardiac monitoring, labs, serum and urine toxicology, and a drug screen.

An eager group of interns and residents awaited the arrival of the medical specialists to hopefully provide some illumination regarding this mysterious wanderer. Her extensive testing, including the MRIs, was entirely normal, the cardiac workup and labs all perfect as well. Psychiatry deemed her nonsuicidal and stable for discharge and outpatient care, referring her to my office for further investigation.

The list of possible conditions—the differential diagnosis—that can produce such seemingly inexplicable behavior is limited. A common type of seizure disorder known as complex partial epilepsy can produce prolonged staring spells and confusional behavior if left untreated with anti-seizure medication. Its victims may stare blankly and exhibit automatic robotic behavior, such as lip smacking, blinking, hand movements, or even bicycle-like leg motion. But in the grips of such a seizure, one cannot exhibit conscious goal-directed complex behavior like booking a flight online, hailing a cab, or boarding an airplane.

Transient global amnesia (TGA) involves brief confusion and disorientation that usually lasts about an hour and typically involves older people with stroke risk factors like hypertension or diabetes. Still, this was a possible explanation.

Drugs, prescribed or illicit, were clearly not involved here. Jane was not suffering from a brain tumor, and there was no evidence of a stroke. She wasn't psychotic or manic and had no history of any psychiatric disorder. She was a responsible and sensible woman with a career. So what compelled her to wander off without any planning or consideration for her family or job? Was she really just an "irresponsible crazy girl" as one inexperienced medical student confidently proclaimed?

Jane had suffered a traumatic event, the death of her mother. This was her first real experience with loss (apart from the death of some family pets over the years). Emotional trauma, especially if sudden, can affect how we process and encode memory. Fear, anger, and sadness can cause mismatching of the neural circuitry that mediates attention span and recall. Somehow, in the grieving and traumatized mind, the hippocampi (which store memories in the right and left temporal lobes) and the amygdalae (which mediate emotions, especially fear, also in the temporal lobes) may become partially "split" or dissociate and fail to network properly. The dramatic result is a zombie-like person who temporarily may engage in seemingly normal and voluntary behavior but in a semiconscious state. This is the so-called fugue or dissociative state. And it can last for days.

Although still grieving the loss of her mother, Jane had seemingly returned to normal daily life by the time she visited my office. She was taking a mild antidepressant medication prescribed by the psychiatrist. She was starting to enjoy her students again and was even considering another Caribbean trip in about a year or so.

"This time, it will be a 'scheduled trip'," she said, using air quotes again. "I think I'm getting docked pay for this last excursion!" We both laughed.

Mrs. Goldberg's Office Visit
or
A Fourteen-Billion-Year History of the Human Brain

It was the end of a long day in the office: three epilepsy patients, five migraine sufferers, a youngish man with Parkinson's, a couple of multiple sclerosis patients, and assorted other mundane and bizarre cases: dizziness, numbness, a young woman who developed amnesia while jogging. And then there was Mrs. Goldberg.

A long-standing patient of mine, Mrs. Goldberg was in her early seventies, a grandmother and housewife. Over the years she underwent multiple neurological workups for a myriad of symptoms, including headaches, dizziness, vertigo, twitching, memory issues, numbness and tingling, faintness, palpitations, decreased taste and smell, and general fatigue. Investigations such as MRIs, EEGs, blood work, second opinions, and third opinions never uncovered any identifiable disorder. By all means she was rather healthy but did suffer some depression and anxiety for which she took medication prescribed by her family physician. Her visits to me at this point were perfunctory. She would tell me about recent events, enumerate new and old symptoms, and wait to be reassured, which I always did, that she was not developing Alzheimer's or some other dreadful disease. She was, in all truth and without condescension, a classic hypochondriac, but a very endearing one.

On one visit, she belabored the issue of how she may have confused a noodle kugel recipe, a beloved Jewish favorite that had been in her family for generations.

"I just don't know what got into me. I overcooked the noodles and added too much cottage cheese. No one really noticed, but I knew something was wrong. After all these years, how could I make such a blunder?" she said, her accent unmistakably Brooklyn and ethnic.

"Mrs. Goldberg, this doesn't mean you are becoming demented. Maybe you were just a little preoccupied or tired," I tried to reassure her.

"No, you don't understand! That's impossible. Cooking noodle kugel is as natural as breathing to me. I've been doing it for decades. No, something is wrong, maybe a brain tumor or a stroke. I need an MRI!"

"Mrs. Goldberg, you just had one a few months ago for those headaches of yours, remember? It was totally normal," I responded.

"Well, you know what I read; yes, I read in the AARP magazine that's just how it starts. First it's the noodle kugel recipe, and before you know it you're in a nursing home, huddled in a corner, and you don't even recognize yourself in the mirror. It's horrible; maybe I should take more vitamins, maybe eat more fish, maybe if I…" She was relentless.

My mind began to wander…

The human brain is about fourteen billion years in the making. A hundred billion neurons with trillions of connections between them, forged from the very atoms that owe their birth to the Big Bang.

Mrs. Goldberg's voice became more distant like she was shrinking…

Fourteen billion years ago, there was nothing—no space, no time, no matter, no energy. Nothing existed except a so-called singularity the size of a period on this page. According to modern science, the singularity contained nearly infinite energy. Then one day, well, so to speak as there were no "days" back then, the singularity exploded releasing matter and energy that inflated throughout the newly formed space and filled it with the first light of photons, then atoms. All the atoms that make up everything in the universe—flowers, computers, baseballs, brains, and people—formed in that early era.

During its first billion years, the universe continued to

expand and cool, and large clumps of matter gravitated to form the one hundred billion galaxies that make up our observable universe. Each of these "island universes," including our Milky Way galaxy, contains about a hundred billion stars. Each of these stars, including our sun, is a thermonuclear furnace. With enough heat and pressure, some of these stars can use the alchemy of fusion to manufacture elements such as carbon, nitrogen, and iron. These are the building blocks of life, but they would be forever useless if they remained locked inside the cores of these great suns. Some of these stars explode as supernovas, among the most luminous objects in the interstellar night. With this fiery death, they spew their life-building elements throughout the galaxy, the star stuff that makes up our very brains and bodies.

About seven billion years ago, an average star was born in a typical spiral galaxy in an ordinary part of the universe. This was our sun in our home galaxy. The gas cloud from which the sun was formed contained enough heavy elements to form the planets, asteroids, and comets that make up our solar system. Our earth formed just at the perfect position, not too far from the sun where liquid oceans would have frozen and not too close where water would vaporize. With just the right "Goldilocks position" from the sun and sufficient atmosphere, the crucial ingredient for life—liquid water—could safely exist.

Perhaps three and a half billion years ago, Promethean-like electrical thunderbolts sparked these chemically rich oceans. The primordial soup was able to produce self-replicating molecules out of amino acids. Simple anaerobic (do not need oxygen to survive) bacteria eventually emerged and transformed earth's carbon dioxide-rich atmosphere into an oxygen-containing one, setting the stage for the evolution of the magnificent diversity of life.

It took two and a half billion years for life to evolve from the earliest cells to multicellular creatures. It took another billion years for fish, amphibians, reptiles, and mammals to emerge. But as the tempo of evolution accelerated, it would only take another hundred million years for our earliest mammalian ancestor—an insect-eating, rat-sized creature—to make its appearance. Six million years ago our chimpanzee relatives, with whom we share 95 percent of our DNA, diverged into the first hominid (our primate and human ancestors) line. The Australopithecus emerged from this branch in the evolutionary tree four million years ago, leaving the dark forest for the bright, sunlit savanna.

A million years ago, the early hominids spread out of Africa and began a great diaspora, entering Asia and Europe. Human brains reached modern-day size about a hundred thousand years ago. At fifty thousand years, all the unique capacities of the human brain were being forged: foresight, imagination, language, and self-awareness.

We are starting to understand the human brain as the product of billions of years of evolution. Natural selection, gene shuffling, and inheritance of traits that increase survivability are all responsible for the painfully slow, incremental changes that have resulted in the remarkable powers of the mind—consciousness, memory, language, and emotions.

Leaving the edge of the solar system and bracing for the long interstellar night, the Voyager 2 spacecraft represents an extension of our collective mind. Launched in 1977, it contains a phonograph of human sounds (greetings in over fifty languages and musical samples ranging from Bach to Chuck Berry) and a recorded message, as well as scientific symbols and notations that presumably could be deciphered by an alien intelligence. This lonely explorer was hurtled into deep space as a cosmic greeting where it may roam, barring some astronomical accident like an asteroid collision, for billions of years. Its epic journey was propelled by one simple question: are we alone in the universe? Are there other minds out there? What really presupposes these mysteries is even one grander query: Is consciousness a cosmic accident unique to the chain of evolutionary events on earth, never to be repeated? Or are there perhaps countless other civilizations in the universe, some thousands or millions of years advanced beyond humanity, doing things and thinking things with their minds that are unimaginable to us?

There is a scientific way of addressing these wondrous musings, and it's called the Drake Equation (named after the astronomer who created it, Frank Drake, one of the pioneers of the Search for Extraterrestrial Intelligence (SETI) movement). The formula involves the following variables: (1) the number of stars in our galaxy that survive long enough for intelligent life to evolve on them, (2) the average number of planets around each of these stars, (3) the fraction of these planets with suitable conditions for life as we know it, and (4) the fraction of these planets that actually produce intelligent civilization, i.e., brains that are intelligent, self-aware, and able to communicate.

Depending on your assumptions—like the probability of life evolving far enough on a planet to produce conscious, intelligent beings, which is anyone's guess—the total number of technologically proficient civilizations just in the Milky Way galaxy could be thousands or millions. Some of these civilizations may be advanced beyond our wildest imagination. It seems statistically likely, at least, that intelligent life has evolved many times over just in our hometown galaxy. Next time you peer into the majestic nighttime sky, remember that knowing eyes and minds may be peering back.

How did we, and our big brains, make it this far? Three and a half billion years ago, radioactive heat warmed a young planet, third from the sun. The first continents started rising above the ancient seas, which were rich in organic molecules like amino acids. One night an electrical discharge from the energized atmosphere, or perhaps the heat from a volcanic eruption, jolted these molecules to self-assemble into tine spheres. These were the first cells, microscopic chemical factories that contain DNA. They self-replicated and ultimately formed what we know today as blue-green algae, paving the way for life beyond the seas.

Colonies of cells set the stage for the development of multicellular creatures like worms and jellyfish. Over the next few millions of years they ruled the oceans, and over the next billion years the first animals with external skeletons—starfish, corals, trilobites—developed. And then fish followed with their spines and separate small brains. In another billion years, man would collect their fossils.

The earth's landscape was still a violent and hostile place at this time. Continents were pushing themselves up through shallow seas while volcanoes erupted. Maybe driven by competition for food, some adventurous fish were pushed to the shoreline and migrated to ponds and streams, and over countess eons they developed lungs for gulping the precious, newly minted oxygen in the atmosphere. These changes in the fish body evolved at an unimaginably slow pace over millions of years.

These air-breathing creatures had better survivability and an improved chance of reproducing. Accidental genetic variations among individual creatures provided the raw genetic material for evolution. And those creatures with the best trait to survive in the current environment were the winners who would reproduce and pass on those traits. Chance and circumstance were the main themes of the evolution of life on earth.

These air-gulping pioneers lived over three hundred million years ago. Tens of millions of generations later these fish developed limbs and started to walk the earth. From these amphibious frogs, another race of creatures would develop.

Two hundred million years ago a great ice age was ending and steamy jungles were covering Asia, Europe, and the Americas. A verdant eden was emerging, but not for humankind. This was the age of the reptiles.

For the next hundred million years, the reptiles ruled this paradise. The most spectacular ones, the dinosaurs, were dull witted but deadly predators like the tyrannosaurus rex or lumbering vegetarians like the brontosaurus. They got by on their instincts alone. The versatility of intelligence was not necessary in their lush world with plenty of food as they were under no pressure to evolve bigger brains. Instinct without intelligence can sometimes get you very far—just look at the insect world with its millions of different species, some of them around unchanged for nearly a billion years.

But by sixty million years ago, something big happened, probably an asteroid collision right into the Yucatan peninsula in what is now Mexico. The climate cooled and the cold-blooded reptiles could not adapt. A random, astronomical catastrophe wiped out the age of the dinosaurs and set the stage for the next chapter in the evolution of life.

Creatures of the night would inherit the earth. When the great lizards walked the earth, these tiny, furry, wide-eyed animals remained nocturnal, subsisting on a diet mainly of insects. They were warm-blooded and could better handle the cooling environment. They resembled, virtually unchanged, the modern tree shrews that you can see at most zoos.

Some of our distant ancestors left the forest floor and

reached for the stars, or at least the tree tops. These tree dwellers were the forerunners of the primates, the ancestors of humans. The evolutionary traits they developed were very different from the ones possessed by the insect-gnawing shrews. The tree dwellers needed a hand, rather than a paw, to grasp branches as they swung precariously high in the forest canopy. They needed stereoscopic vision to accurately judge distances and color vision to detect the brightly colored fruits against the green forest background, as well as noticing camouflaged predators in the shadows. These traits would confer greatly improved survivability on those who inherited them.

The brain of the tree dwellers got bigger and more complex, and after about thirty million years, according to the fossil record, they morphed into another kind of creature, the monkey. As these delicate tree-swinging primates evolved, they became sturdier and stronger apes and ultimately left the seclusion of the forest for the open grasslands.

Australopithecus, the ape hominid, arrived on the scene about four million years ago. She (our most complete fossil skeleton is that of the female named "Lucy") walked on two legs (bipedal) and used her free hands to forage for fruits, nuts, and insects; made primitive stone flakes; and lived in the open savannas.

Homo habilis ("handyman") and Homo erectus eventually evolved from Lucy's descendants. These hominids fashioned choppers, scrapers, and flakes, and they used these tools to hunt and cut meat from the calorie-rich marrow of the animal bones.

Bigger brains with more elaborate neural circuitry needed more energy to operate. Foresight, planning, and imagination were now part of the evolving cerebral cortex. The "big bang" in brain size had already started. Bipedalism, a finely skilled pair of hands, and stereoscopic color vision all set the stage for human culture, science, and technology. And the great "out of Africa" exodus began as our descendents migrated to Asia and Indonesia.

By a million years ago, we were probably hunting in groups and communicating with guttural sounds. The Neanderthal man became a skilled hunter and cave dweller by 150,000 years ago and probably broke the long loneliness with complex speech. But these hardy ancestors were ultimately replaced by our very own Homo sapiens. These men and women were great adventurers and migrated to Europe and even crossed the open ocean to reach Australia by 40,000 years ago. They left behind a legacy of hauntingly beautiful cave paintings, hearths, and polished tools. They fashioned flutes out of ivory and Venus figurines—naked women amulets out of stone. The name given to this era by modern-day humans is the Paleolithic or Human Revolution.

Some day this great creature, who sixty million years ago was a lonely and frightened tree shrew hiding in the dark, would build great telescopes to study the heavens, devise machines to peer into his body and brain, and threaten his very existence with atomic weapons. He would be the only species on the planet to wonder about his place in the universe.

"Dr. Adamo, are you listening? I don't believe you've heard a word I've said!" Mrs. Goldberg must have noticed my momentary inattentiveness.

"Of course I am, Mrs. Goldberg. You were saying…ah yes, the noodle kugel recipe," I confidently replied.

"No, no, no, that was five minutes ago. I'm wondering about the vitamins. Should I be taking extra B12, thiamine, folate? And what about ginkgo and that jellyfish protein they always advertise on TV for memory and to focus better?"

"Oh, yes, let's discuss that," I quickly answered, trying to appear ready to delve into her questions with some feigned enthusiasm. "But please forgive me, Mrs. Goldberg, sometimes my mind wanders too…"

Memories of Dreams

Dreams have captured the wonderment of humans for millennia. The ancient Paleolithic caves at Lascaux and Altamira depict beautiful, surrealistic images that may represent dreamy recollections of the hunt. The Sumerians in Mesopotamia, as well as the Greeks, viewed dreams as prophecies and omens, full of hidden meanings and warnings. In the Judeo-Christian heritage, dreams represent the voice of the one God. The Hindus tell us that the dream state is just one of the three realms of being, along with wakefulness and sleep. Freud called dreams the "royal road to the unconscious." In his revolutionary view, dreams contained all the symbolism that represents the hidden fears and desires of the unconscious mind. Modern neurology analyzes dreams in terms of neurophysiologic brain states. During the REM sleep state, characterized by rapid eye movement and loss of body muscle tone, the brain seems to be electrically almost awake. Most dreams and nightmares occur at this stage but may also occur less frequently during the alternating non-REM stages. Most dreams are forgotten or remembered only in fragments, but some memories of dreams are as vivid as real experiences.

Over the years, there have been some who have confided such memories to me, perhaps in the hopes that it would be of some medical benefit or perhaps just out of the desire to share a private or painful experience.

"It was a big colonial farmhouse on Iowa farmland. I spent the first twenty years of my life there. It sat on an open plain, back in Iowa, built by my grandparents. I eventually moved only because I got married and my husband had business back in New York," Joan explained when I queried about where she grew up and the origin of her Midwestern twang. Widowed, she was an inveterate insomniac, even now with the worries of raising a family long in the past. She enjoyed her grandchildren and good health but still could never sleep well. She underwent complete polysomnography studies: wired up with brain wave, cardiac, breathing, and movement monitors overnight in a hospital sleep lab. No sleep apnea was detected, no seizure activity, and no heart arrhythmias. REM and non-REM sleep stages were nicely proportioned throughout the evening. And Joan even slept most of the night, an unusual feat under the uncomfortable circumstances of the sleep lab.

"Your study is very normal," I explained. "Often, primary insomnia goes unexplained with no discernible disorder evident. Sometimes it's easy. We often see evidence of disrupted sleep, sleep apnea, RLS (restless leg syndrome), REM sleep disorder, nocturnal seizures. But in your case, nothing's obvious here. Do you have dreams or nightmares?"

"Well, I wouldn't call it a nightmare, but I do have a recurring dream, on and off for years now."

"What about taking an occasional drug? There are several sedative-hypnotics that we could try in low dose. They're often used for persistent insomnia."

"No, Doc. I already tried a few of them—Ambien, Restoril, and Klonopin. Sometimes they worked, but they stopped my dreams, and in the morning I would feel tired anyway. There's been this recurrent dream and, well, I kind of look forward to having it. It's been going on for years now."

"Is it a nightmare?" I asked.

"No, it's a little spooky—haunting, I guess you'd say—but I do kind of enjoy it. And each time I have it, it gets a little clearer and I remember more of it."

"What is it about, your husband?" I suggested.

She sighed and shook her head no. "It's about growing up back in that house in Iowa. It was an immense house, three stories with rooms within rooms. We could play hide-and-seek for hours. There was one room that my siblings and friends usually avoided. The attic was way up, perched on the third floor, and you had to take a fourth fight of rickety steps to reach it, but it was a treasure trove. It seemed like I could spend hours in there just waiting to be found by one of the other children."

I smiled. Joan was nearing eighty, but I could see how she

relished this childhood memory.

She continued, "There was all sorts of stuff up there: old family photos and family portraits, closets full of stylish clothes from the 1900s, old china plates, dolls, wind-up toys, a stuffed bear head that my grandpa had shot. There were boxes of diaries, old books, and an old Bible almost too heavy to lift, an old phonograph that could still play scratchy records of big band music…" She paused and became teary-eyed. "Each night, the dreams become a bit more detailed as if somehow my mind is able to dredge up more details of those many hours I spent in that dark attic, with a lantern in my hand, pouring over old diaries and letters. Letters about foreign lands, a trip to New York City long ago, the wedding of a great aunt I never knew. I don't know if everything I'm remembering in my dreams is true or if my imagination is just filling in the gaps. Either way, I welcome them."

"I don't know, Joan. The mind often fills in those gaps in a biographical narrative, whether it is a real experience or just a dream. That's one reason why recollections, even those of fairly recent events, can be so unreliable. It can be impossible to tell how accurate any memory is, especially memories that manifest in the dream world."

Joan didn't appreciate my medical skepticism. She was like an archaeologist, each night excavating and discovering relics of a lost world and, with those relics, trying to reconstruct an ancient past. A past full of wonder and magic, a past of which she was perhaps the sole survivor.

He was a religious man, raised a strict Irish-Catholic in a working class neighborhood of Queens, New York. For his entire adult life he worked as a fireman and now, after two decades, was about to retire and pursue a second career as a carpenter. He was one of the many heroic 9/11 first responders who watched helplessly as bodies fell from the sky, men and women jumping from a hundred stories up to escape flames and heat, knowing full well that certain death waited below. He and his heroic colleagues ran into the burning towers fully realizing that death would meet many of them as well. Bill the Fireman, as my office staff sometimes affectionately referred to him, survived the catastrophe of the collapsing towers but did suffer complications: asthma-like symptoms—an unexplained cough and mild fatigue—and some mild memory issues. This last symptom was the reason he consulted with me. He also suffered the almost universal malady of adversity victims: post-traumatic stress disorder (PTSD). A good marriage and family life kept his anxiety and depressive symptoms in check. An occasional panic attack was tolerable, and even the recurrent nightmares and flashbacks were tolerable, except for one.

"It goes like this, Dr. A.," he confided to me on his second office visit. "I'm climbing down the stairs of some large building, probably a skyscraper, but it's not the towers, and I'm working my way down endless flights of stairs. On one floor, it's like a vast office or library, and I see Asian people, mostly young, all working at their desks or tables. They're doing calculations; there are books and computers everywhere. I get the feeling they're working urgently against the clock. I pass them by quickly and then reach another floor. This one's like one of those natural history museum dioramas. It seems like I'm outside now. It's nighttime and it's some kind of forest. I think I can see or hear dinosaurs in the distance. The sky is full of stars. There's a house there too—looks like the one I grew up in back in Brooklyn. I try to enter it, but I have to go down the next flight of stairs." He paused and looked at me quizzically.

"I can't possibly tell you what this all means, but it's pretty imaginative," I say with a smile.

"Well, finally I think I reach a basement or bottom floor. The walls are all concrete and seem very heavy. There are corridors everywhere. I can hear murmurs, or maybe faint screams, behind me or above me. I meet my father, who died a few years ago, and he's walking down the corridor. He seems lost or confused and doesn't speak to me; maybe he doesn't even recognize me, but he leads me to a room. I open the door—it's like a doctor's waiting room. There are people sitting along the walls. There's a fireplace that's working, and there is a closed door on each side. I remember thinking that maybe the doors open up to heaven and hell, and that the waiting room is purgatory."

"So what do you do?" I asked, by now thoroughly engrossed.

"Well, nothing because I always wake up before I can decide which door to open."

Christian symbolism, the loss of a parent, busy financial

analysts oblivious to the impending terrorist attack, the grand scheme of life on earth—I had all sorts of interpretations, but I didn't offer any. I'm sure Bill had better ones.

Twentysomething, energetic, and bright, Laura was a newly minted lawyer who'd had epilepsy since childhood. Her seizures were well controlled on one medication, but she could still suffer an occasional brief nocturnal seizure, which her husband typically notified her about the next morning. Her infrequent seizures only occurred during sleep—a few myoclonic jerks of the arms or legs, some stertorous breathing, and it was all over in a few minutes. Often triggered by an occasional alcoholic drink or mild sleep deprivation, they fortunately played no major role in her daily awake life. Sometimes the only telltale sign that one may have occurred was her remembrance of a dream the next morning, a rather elaborate dream that seemed to only occur on those nights when the nocturnal paroxysm paid a visit.

"It's not a nightmare, really. It plays out rather slowly, and I think I usually recall it pretty well by the next morning. In one form or another I've been having this dream for a few years now. It starts where I'm walking toward an older Victorian-style house. There's lots of land around, so I get the impression it's not a suburban area. It's nighttime and there seems to be some kind of social event or reunion party taking place. It looks like there are Christmas lights strung over some of the trees, but it seems to be autumn because I can hear leaves rustling in the surrounding woods. I walk up the porch stairs slowly. Inside there are lots of people and piano music is playing. There are butlers and maids too. People are talking in groups of two or three or four. I'm drawn to the corner of the room where there is a young family, a mom and dad and two kids. I gradually recognize them. It's my family—my parents and my sister when we were about ten years old."

Laura continued to explain, with some emotional intensity, the rest of her dream, or at least her recollection of it. It is always remarkable to me that the remembrance of a dream can carry so much emotional weight; after all, the mind is retracing something that never happened but is rather a figment of its own imagination. And yet, such a memory can be indelibly ingrained with us for all time.

As her adult self realized she was standing next to her younger self, she tried to listen in on her family's conversation but couldn't understand or hear clearly what they were discussing. They seemed curiously oblivious to her, or as she explained, "I felt like I was a ghost, just eavesdropping." Frustrated with this current state of events, she walked on to another part of the enormous ballroom. Next, she encountered a somewhat older version of herself, as well as her parents, and herself and sister, now teenagers. "I knew we were teenagers at this point just by our look and demeanor, and I was wearing a familiar favorite outfit—a denim button-down shirt, jeans, and boots."

She was content just to stand next to her younger parents

and sister, still unable to decipher the conversation, but one of the butlers seemed to motion her through the doorway to the next room.

"It is then that I realized that all the people at this place were mostly family or friends, aunts, cousins, grandparents," Laura said excitedly.

The next room was kind of an open-air garden veranda. She could now see the clear starry sky and still hear the autumn trees rustling in the wind.

Now her parents were older, and Laura saw herself standing with her future fiancé. Finally, someone in the garden seemed to acknowledge her presence, a maid who offered her a glass of wine. She reached for it, but when she turned around to rejoin her family, they had vanished. She hurriedly walked down a garden pathway illuminated with string lights. She noticed an elderly couple, perhaps her parents, walking into the night.

And, Laura explained, "I see a couple with two toddlers, and I'm convinced that this is my future family. My hair is shorter and my husband is a little heavier, and for some strange reason, he's wearing a Yankee's cap—football is his sport, and besides, he's a Red Sox fan having grown up in Boston.

"Before I can try to join them, I'm escorted back out of the house, which is now mostly empty, and I'm led to the front porch again, standing in the cool night air, wishing I could go back in. But the front doors are then closed, and I start to reluctantly walk toward the darkened woods…"

Final Greetings from Room 237

On a bright summer day I was called to consult on a nursing home patient whom I had evaluated a few weeks earlier. Eleanor was a ninety-two-year-old lady who had fairly advanced dementia and had been a resident of the home for about a year. She had raised five children and helped pack artillery shells during World War II. She'd been a widow for over two decades. Her children, except for one daughter, rarely visited her. They gave up when she stopped being able to recognize them. She ate well, walked with some assistance, and cursed out the staff relentlessly, despite their sincerest efforts to mollify her. I was summoned to readjust her medications. The staff was becoming weary of her impudence.

"Eleanor, what's all this trouble you're causing? They tell me you're always yelling at the staff will all manner of profanities. What's wrong?" I asked with a forced smile.

"These goddamn people are a bunch of morons. You know, I coulda been an astronaut; yeah, that's right. But I raised a family. These morons don't know a damn thing. This is my damn house. Who the hell do they think they are, coming and going in and out and all the time?"

"Eleanor, you're in a nursing home. These people are staff members—doctors, nurses, physical therapists. They're here to help you," I responded earnestly.

"Sonny, you seem like a nice enough boy, but you really don't know what the hell you're talking about. Let me tell you, the clock's a ticking away for you too. The good Lord is gonna come calling and take your soul back."

She took a deep breath as if she were mustering all her decaying mind's effort to draw up a memory: "I put together army weapons in Picatinny…but now I can't remember my children's names or faces."

Ultimately, I decided not to increase her sedative medication. The staff would just have to deal with her obnoxiousness. I figured she earned it. As I made my exit, Eleanor, in what was either a moment of brilliant lucidity or demented psychosis, provided me with some chilling advice.

"Sonny, watch for the black dot, the black dot. It's there; it's always there!" she exclaimed.

I briefly wondered if she was experiencing a hallucination or maybe a scotoma-like visual defect, perhaps resulting from her aging retina. But it soon became clear she was speaking metaphorically. Or at least I thought she might be.

"It doesn't matter how blue the sky is. Even on the clearest day, the brightest day, it's there. You can barely see it…but as you get on in years it gets larger, darker. Sooner or later you can't ignore it. Maybe, at first, it's far away, on the horizon. But it's coming, it's coming, coming for you, for all of us—gettin' bigger and bigger until it'll swallow you up—and then that's it; it's all over." She stared intently at the ceiling, but looking beyond it.

I smiled at her. "All right, Eleanor, I'll keep that in mind," I answered patronizingly.

I exited the building and stepped out into the bright midday sun. The azure sky was as clear as I'd ever seen. I gazed up at it but couldn't find a single blemish, cloud or plane. But then, maybe, I caught a glimpse of something on the eastern horizon. A small dot. Probably just a distant aircraft? I quickly averted my gaze and headed home to my family.

Afterlife

Sometimes there is a thin line that separates science and superstition, fact and faith, the known and the unknowable. This is often encountered, especially toward the end of life, in the twilight regions of coma with all its horrid variations: persistent vegetative state, minimally conscious state, locked-in state, and brain death. All of these are often a prelude to what Shakespeare called the "undiscovered country."

Coma is a state of unconsciousness, but unlike sleep it is the result of some type of brain injury- head trauma, a stroke, or cardiac arrest. It may be deep, with no awareness or light, with some arousal or wakefulness. People in deep coma often die. Persistent vegetative state (often abbreviated as PVS in the technical literature) is perhaps the most vexing. After some type of brain injury—often major head trauma in a young person from a motor vehicle accident—a person will lie in a hospital bed, remaining still with eyes open, breathing but with no voluntary movement of limbs, and seemingly no awareness of self or the environment. It is a cruel fate, as often families cannot accept the painful fact that these victims will never wake up although they appear awake. Sometimes coma victims start to exhibit improvement—they may follow simple verbal commands, have voluntary movements, and make gestures, even speaking one- or two-word responses. Such a minimally conscious state (MCS) shows hopeful improvement but typically does not result in any major recovery.

Locked-in syndrome is different. Often the result of a large brain-stem stroke, the victim is totally paralyzed and mute but with completely preserved cognitive function. Awake and fully alert, they can communicate using alphabet boards, eye movements, and eye blinks, and possess as rich a language and intellectual function as anyone (the book *The Diving Bell and the Butterfly* was remarkably composed by such a person while in a locked-in state).

Then there is brain death. Imagine a woman lying in an intensive care unit bed. She recently had a massive stroke or perhaps cardiac arrest at home. She is silent; a ventilator inflates and deflates her lungs with oxygen. Intravenous medications maintain her heart rate and blood pressure. Her skin is warm and sweaty. Yet there is no limb movement; she is totally unresponsive and unarousable. Even primitive reflexes such as throat gag, eye blinks, or pupillary responses cannot be elicited. Ultimately she may be declared brain dead, indicating the irreversible and catastrophic loss of all brain function with no prospect of any recovery. Brain death is recognized legally as death because we recognize that a heart kept pumping by drugs and mechanically inflated lungs without a functioning brain is not life. The painful paradox is the brain dead appear only to be in a coma, but brain death is not coma, deep or otherwise.

Which brings us to OBL, which we would eventually (and affectionately) call a grandmother who found herself in the ICU one Saturday evening. She was cleaning up her backyard after a busy summer day enjoying her grandchildren. Her waterfront home was bathed in the golden light of the sunset as she picked up the inflatable water toys, Frisbees, and beach balls. She felt a sudden loss of breath and later recalled to me that her heart felt like "a galloping racehorse." She collapsed onto the manicured green lawn. Her daughter ran toward her and wisely started CPR but stopped after a few chest compressions when she realized her mother was breathing on her own. Since the grandmother resided just a few life-saving minutes down the road from the hospital, she arrived in the ER soon after 911 was called.

It was promptly determined that she had suffered a fairly large heart attack. By the time she was in the ER, she had regained full alertness and was able to speak, but she still was a bit bewildered by this quick, unfortunate turn of events on an otherwise perfect day. Although fragile and elderly, she gradually gained enough strength to undergo a cardiac angiogram a few days later, and stents were placed in two of her blocked heart arteries. She jovially referred to her cardiac procedure as "just your basic plumbing job unclogging a few of the old lady's pipes."

While convalescing in intensive care I was asked to see her—just a routine consult to assess her neurological condition after suffering a brief but nearly disastrous cardiac arrest. She was witty and sharp. Her amnestic period for the episode was minimal: she recalled most of the day with her grandchildren, picking up toys on the lawn, and partially recalled the ambulance ride. Rather impressive, I thought, as often memory for the entire day or more may be wiped out in such circumstances, to say nothing of more severe traumatic brain injury.

On the hospital cart next her bed was what a cursory observer might mistake for a game board. It was flat, wooden, chipped, and weatherworn. It had the letters of the alphabet, numbers zero through nine, the words "yes," "no," "hello," and "goodbye," along with some symbols—a half moon, a five-pointed star, and a circle. A separate heart-shaped wooden piece (which I would later learn is called a planchette), just small enough to fit in the palm, sat on top of the board.

I stared at it; my curiosity must have seemed obvious.

"That's my Ouija board, Doctor. Ever seen one?" she asked plainly.

"Oh yes, the last time I did was as a kid. There was a time when they were as popular as Monopoly, but why do you have one?"

"I've had this one since I was a child. Always liked playing with it. I'm a devout Catholic, so I don't give much credence to supernatural gibberish, but who knows? A few times over the years it's guessed right. My mother despised it, thought it was the devil's work."

The Ouija board, I reviewed later that evening, gained popularity here in America after the Civil War, as the spiritualist movement grew. People consulted mediums in the hope of communicating with dead relatives. Necromancy via Ouija boards became a popular commercial parlor game. Hasbro (yes, that Hasbro) eventually became the biggest manufacturer of the board/planchette combo.

I remember, as a skeptical but inquisitive kid, asking the board questions such as "Who killed JFK?" and "Will I go to heaven or hell?" The most aggressive player with the strongest fingers, it seemed, would always manage to spell out his or her message.

There is, however, a neurological explanation for this supernatural chicanery. Participants in the game, especially if they are true believers, may put themselves into a kind of dissociative state where their actions—spelling out a desired message they believe is being transmitted from a loved one in the great beyond—are automatic or semi-unconscious. The player becomes so emotionally worked up during a séance that they are not fully cognizant of moving the planchette and spelling out their desired message. The phenomenon called "facilitated communication" presents a similar scenario. Eager parents "guide" the hands of a severely autistic child along a keyboard resulting in impossible literary biographies full of nuanced emotion. Shining a light of detached objectivity onto these cases clearly demonstrates that the parents, not the impaired child, are desperately writing and projecting their own stories either consciously or unconsciously. Is there a stronger force in nature than a parent's love of his or her child? For that matter, is there a stronger force than love of anything or anyone?

Ouija Board Lady did well during the ensuing days, despite her recent heart attack. Her board game was a hit with the medical staff. The nurses, physical therapists, and resident physicians, all young adults just starting off in their lives and careers, took a real liking to her and often would participate in a brief session. They would pose such questions as "Who will I marry?" and "Will I live a long life?" and "How is my aunt Terry doing?" to which OBL would judiciously engage her mysterious plank of wood and come up with the answers: "Your frog will be your prince" and "You will live as long as necessary" and "Your aunt is alive but not well; you should call her!" (It turned out to be a surprisingly relevant response.) Some took her seriously, but most simply enjoyed her maternal good-natured way. It was always hard to tell if she really took herself and her Ouija board seriously.

One evening, just four days after her admission, she suffered another cardiac event: a brief run of ventricular tachycardia, perhaps the most life-threatening of all heart arrhythmias. She became unconscious, and a code was called—CPR started, IV meds—and just after about forty-five seconds, as the anesthesiologist was ready to intubate and place her on a life-support ventilator, she came to. Her eyes opened, and she was able to utter some appropriate words. Our ninety-year-old OBL had escaped her demise a second time.

I was asked to see her the next day—a typical consult request after any patient suffers a near-fatal event—to assess any neurological impairment that may have resulted from her second cardiac event.

"How are you feeling?" I asked, trying to play down the fact that the day before she almost died.

"I think I'm okay, just feel a little winded. The cardiologist says that's normal after what happened."

"You look good to me. Any trouble with your memory or trouble finding words?"

"None that I can tell."

I smiled. "Where's your trusty partner (referring to her Ouija board)?"

"Well, I haven't been toying with it…you know, I had some kind of weird dream yesterday when I passed out. I was standing in the corner over there"—she motioned to the right side of the room near the window—"It was like I was watching the doctors work on me—the nurses, the internist—and then I realized my husband and my sister were standing next to me clear as day. I haven't seen either of them in over a decade; they both passed. My husband touched my shoulder and smiled…" Her eyes watered.

NDEs, I explained, are common after a life-threatening medical event such as a heart attack. Survivors of near-death experiences often recount certain universal themes: out-of-body sensation or floating through a dark tunnel to a bright light; meeting loved ones, living or dead; jarring Proustian recollection of life experiences or an entire lifetime in a fleeting instant. People report a sense of something numinous, divine, or awe-inspiring. Some near-death experiences, however, are frightening with a sense of terror or loneliness. In all cases they are vividly recollected.

On a psychological level, none of this is surprising. A brush with death reminds us of the fragile and precarious grip we have on our transient earthly stay. We are forced to realize our mortality without any elaborate denial. On a neurological level, the hypoxia (lack of oxygen) and ischemia (lack of blood flow) that occur during a catastrophic event, such as stroke or cardiac arrest, results in sudden and dramatic changes in brain physiology. The fuel-starved brain with its electrically misfiring neurons creates a firestorm, perhaps a type of seizure or lucid dream. The dying brain constructs one final narrative—a story of our personal heaven or hell, a fleeting visit to an afterlife, the undiscovered country, the transition from life to oblivion.

Our Ouija Board Lady, however, had a different explanation: "I think it was a glimpse, Doc, a glimpse of maybe what comes next."

Three nights later, resting comfortably in the step-down cardiac unit, she suffered her final cardiac arrest. She had been doing well, tenacious and independent, and there was talk of transferring her to cardiac rehab and then home. The night nurse was enjoying a game of Ouija board with her, posing queries like "Who will win the next presidential election?" and "What part of the world will my great-grandchildren live?"

But the heart monitor alerted another run of ventricular tachycardia, this time sustained, and a full code was conducted, which dutifully included CPR, intubation, and a hook-up to a mechanical respirator. The code lasted twenty minutes.

Each of us will die one day. It is an inevitable and immutable consequence of life. The physicists tell us it's simply the result of thermodynamics—the flow of entropy and the ultimate breakdown of everything. Someday, perhaps, through some remotely advanced technology, humans or our distant descendants may become immortal, but for us, barring a real afterlife of some kind, there is no such luck. Humans have developed a few coping mechanisms for this haunting reality. The first is simple denial: we turn away from it, create families, find meaning in our work, get check-ups, jump on the treadmill, and take vitamins. This is the foundation of civilization; we do not live in despair of the inevitable but forge ahead. Religion provides the second means of eradicating our fear of ultimate oblivion. The Judeo-Christian heaven promises us eternal life. Buddhism gives us the eternal cycle of reincarnation. The modern transhumanism (or techno-humanism) movement hopes for a kind of "digital rapture" where we all upload our minds to the Cloud (or replace our frail carbon-based bodies with something more durable).

I would be called to reevaluate OBL a couple of days later. She appeared to be in deep irreversible coma, perhaps brain death, and as the neurologist of record, I was asked to address this issue with the ICU staff and family.

The concept of brain death, death as a sort of irreversible coma with total loss of brain function, developed decades ago when it became possible to resuscitate people through CPR and mechanical ventilation (respirators). This typically occurs in hospitals, as most deaths occur after one's heart stops beating, breathing stops, and the body and brain die together. In brain death, however, the body still functions. The chest rises and falls with artificial breaths, the heart beats, the body perspires, and fingernails grow. Pregnant young mothers, brain dead for weeks, have given birth to viable babies.

It strains credulity to convince families that their loved one, who appears to be resting comfortably, is dead.

"Quite simply, we know that when your brain is dead, you are dead," I explained bluntly to the children and grandchildren surrounding the ICU bed. "Her heart and lungs are being forced to function now, only to send blood and oxygen to a brain that has been destroyed. Everything we know tells us that even her most primitive brain-stem functions, including independent breathing, have permanently ceased. As a result, her consciousness, personality, memories, and emotional capacity have all been eradicated as well." I silently scolded myself. I should have been more aggressive about obtaining a DNR (do not resuscitate) order earlier; the family could have been spared this ordeal.

"What about a brain CT or EEG? I read that those are important tests," one of her eager grandchildren, a nurse, asked me.

"Such tests are unnecessary at this point," I responded simply, sensing that the family was beginning to understand the futility of the situation. Shudder the thought of performing an EEG on this poor lady. We know that brain wave activity is entirely absent in brain death, so-called flat line or isoelectric. Years ago, as an overly zealous attempt to convince a family member of the diagnosis, I had one performed in the ICU on a similar but younger patient. The electrical artifact of the ICU (produced by the whirling activity of respirators, IV machines, and cardiac monitors all running continuous electrical current) produced a weird sinusoidal wave form on the brain wave tracing. It was clearly artifactual but enough to sadly convince the family that their loved one was misdiagnosed and would wake up. He didn't.

The family allowed our Ouija Board Lady to be disconnected a few hours later. Because she was too old to harvest viable organs from, they asked that her body be donated to a medical school. They saw how admired she was by the young medical staff. They thought she would have wanted this. They remembered her words: "The soul goes wherever it is that souls go; the body stays here forever."

www.ingramcontent.com/pod-product-compliance
Lightning Source LLC
Chambersburg PA
CBHW020634220526
45464CB00001B/150